Manual of

Manual of
ULTRASOUND

Third Edition

GS Garkal MBBS DMRD MD

Consultant Radiologist
Janta X-ray Clinic Laboratory Pvt Ltd
New Delhi, India

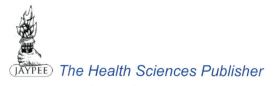

The Health Sciences Publisher

New Delhi | London | Philadelphia | Panama

Jaypee Brothers Medical Publishers (P) Ltd.

Headquarters
Jaypee Brothers Medical Publishers (P) Ltd.
4838/24, Ansari Road, Daryaganj
New Delhi 110 002, India
Phone: +91-11-43574357
Fax: +91-11-43574314
E-mail: jaypee@jaypeebrothers.com

Overseas Offices

J.P. Medical Ltd.
83, Victoria Street, London
SW1H 0HW (UK)
Phone: +44-20 3170 8910
Fax: +44(0) 20 3008 6180
E-mail: info@jpmedpub.com

Jaypee-Highlights Medical Publishers Inc.
City of Knowledge, Building 235, 2nd Floor
Clayton, Panama City, Panama
Phone: +1 507-301-0496
Fax: +1 507-301-0499
E-mail: cservice@jphmedical.com

Jaypee Medical Inc.
325, Chestnut Street
Suite 412, Philadelphia, PA 19106, USA
Phone: +1 267-519-9789
E-mail: support@jpmedus.com

Jaypee Brothers Medical Publishers (P) Ltd.
17/1-B, Babar Road, Block-B, Shaymali
Mohammadpur, Dhaka-1207
Bangladesh
Mobile: +08801912003485
E-mail: jaypeedhaka@gmail.com

Jaypee Brothers Medical Publishers (P) Ltd.
Bhotahity, Kathmandu, Nepal
Phone: +977-9741283608
E-mail: kathmandu@jaypeebrothers.com

Website: www.jaypeebrothers.com
Website: www.jaypeedigital.com

Manual of Ultrasound

First Edition: 1992
Second Edition: 2002
Third Edition: 2017

ISBN: 978-93-5250-123-6

Printed at Rajkamal Electric Press, Plot No. 2, Phase-IV, Kundli, Haryana.

Dedicated to

Dr Protima Garkal

Preface to the Third Edition

The purpose of writing this third edition book is to provide a thoroughly revised and updated book to the readers and to add a chapter of basic sonography of soft tissue.

I am thankful to Ms Sonia Thakur (Professional Assistant) for her help in completion of this book.

Finally, I am thankful to Dr Protima Garkal for encouraging me to update the book.

Before concluding, I further desire to acknowledge my great indebtedness to Shri Jitendar P Vij (Group Chairman), Mr Ankit Vij (Group President), Mr Tarun Duneja (Director–Publishing), Mr KK Raman (Production Manager), and staff of M/s Jaypee Brothers Medical Publishers (P) Ltd, New Delhi, India, for publishing the book.

GS Garkal

Preface to the First Edition

In accordance with wishes of private practitioners, this book has been written chiefly for the people who are interested in becoming Ultrasonographer and Ultrasonologist in X-ray and ultrasound clinics. I feel even the doctors and unit incharges who possess ultrasound units but are not radiologists can also be benefited significantly.

I must admit that in the preparation of the book, I have freely consulted various books and periodicals, to the authors of which I acknowledge my grateful thanks.

I express my sincere thanks to Drs RK Jain and Mukul Jain, Chikitsa Nursing Home, Saket, New Delhi, India, for every possible assistance to facilitate the completion of book.

I also express my sincere gratitude to Mr RK Verma (Radiographer), Chikitsa Nursing Home, and Miss Anita Arora (Receptionist and Typist) Anupam Diagnostic Centre, Shalimar Bagh, New Delhi for typing of the book.

Finally, I am also thankful to Drs (Mrs) Yash Bhagra, SP Gupta, Shyam Gupta and Kulbir Handa, for encouraging me in writing the book.

GS Garkal

Contents

1

Basic Principles of Ultrasound

What is ultrasound? It may be defined as waves of sound beyond the ordinary limits of hearing. Therefore, simplified to high-frequency sound waves, sound waves are a vibratory phenomenon and they require matter for their transmission. Sound also travels best in substances composed of many molecules therefore, it will travel better through solids composed of multiple molecules than it will in gases such as air, in which there are fewer molecules. For our purposes, we will limit our discussion of sound waves to high-frequency waves since these are the type used in medical diagnosis.

Unlike audible sound, high-frequency sound can be directed in a beam (much like light) and in so doing follows the laws of reflection and refraction, making it possible to reflect off objects of very small size. The main disadvantage of high-frequency sound is that it travels poorly through air, requiring an airless contact with the body during examination. This explains the need to use mineral oil or jelly as a coupling agent to body areas being examined.

Sound is actually a series of compressions and rarefactions. The combination of one compression and one rarefaction represents one cycle. The distance between one cycle and the onset of next cycle is the wave length (λ). The speed at which sound travels through a given medium is its velocity. Now, we can define frequency as the number of cycles over a given period of time. Therefore, the velocity is equal to the frequency multiplied by the wavelength ($V = F \times \lambda$). By this equation, you can see that frequency and wavelength are inversely related. The higher is the frequency, and the smaller is the wavelength.

How sound travels through a medium is often referred to as the *acoustic impedance* of that medium. For example, as sound travels through the bladder it is going in essentially a straight line. When it reaches an interface (or border) between the bladder and the uterus, a portion of the beam is reflected or refracted back to the transducer while the majority of the beam continues in a straight line through the body.

Ultrasound with a higher frequency (or smaller wavelength) can reflect sound from smaller objects, since a higher frequency ultrasound beam has greater *resolution*. Resolution is the ability to visualize objects of interfaces close to one another. For example, the transducer used most often in abdominal and obstetrical sonography is the 2.25 or 3.5 MHz transducer, because the average depth of the area of interest in this case is 20–40 cm. However, in scanning the thyroid, (which is usually less than 7 cm away from the transducer) a 10 MHz transducer is better since it sacrifices depth for better resolution or detail nearer the surface.

The area closest to the transducer is termed the *near field* and that farthest away, the *far field*. The ultrasound beam encounters numerous interfaces on its path through the body. At each of these interfaces, part of the sound beam is reflected back and a smaller portion passes through the interface. This diminishes the sonic beam and leaves progressively less and less available for deep penetration. In addition to the reflection of the sound beam there is also sonic *absorption* and *scatter*, causing even more weakening of the sonic beam. This phenomenon is referred to as attenuation of the sound beam. A term used to express the amount of absorption and attenuation of the sound beam is *half value layer*. This term may be defined as the distance sound will travel in a given medium before its energy is attenuated one half its original value. The fluid and homogenous tissue are excellent conductors of sound while bone has a very low half value layer, presenting a veritable barrier to the sonic beam.

The velocity (speed) of sound depends on the density and elasticity of the medium through which it travels. Velocity also depends on temperature of the medium. However, since the human body temperature is relatively constant, temperature changes are not usually important in medical diagnostic work. The velocity of sound through living human soft tissue is 1540 m/s. The only significant change of velocity encountered by the ultrasound beam would be as it traveled through gas or bone. The greater the acoustic difference, the more sound will be reflected back to the transducer. Another important factor governing the amount of sound reflected is the angle at which the beam strikes the interface (angle of incidence). The closer the angle of incidence is to 90° to the interface, the more the sound is reflected.

Ultrasound Instruments

Components of an Echograph

Acoustic imaging depends primarily on the property of reflection together with pulsing of the beam. Electrical energy is intermittently fed into the transducer, so that the crystal emits short bursts of sound (less than one millisecond in duration). Following this emission, the transducer is quiescent, acting as a receiver (99 milliseconds duration) for any reflected sound waves or echoes. The rate at which the sound is pulsed into the body is called the *repetition rate* (Fig. 2.1).

Signal Processing

When the reflected sound beam returns to the transducer, an electrical impulse is created and transmitted back to the ultrasound machine (echograph). This impulse is in the form of a radio frequency or RF signal, and is seen as a burst of echoes rising above or below the baseline. However, before this RF signal is allowed to print on the CRT (cathode ray tube), it is electronically processed, so that only the envelope or upper half of the signal is presented on the face of the oscilloscope screen.

Transducers

Ultrasonic waves used in medical diagnosis are generated by a *transducer*. The currently used transducers are made from man-made crystals such as

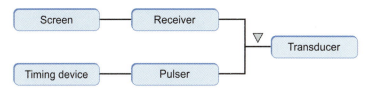

Fig. 2.1 Components of an echograph

barium titanate and lead zirconate. These elements were selected because of their piezoelectric qualities. Piezoelectricity can be defined as a pressure electric effect, i.e. when a substance changes shape under the influence of an electric field. The Curie Brothers first noted the piezoelectric effect when they found that if an electrical current was sent through a quartz crystal, the shape of the crystal would vary with the polarity. As the crystal expands and contracts it produces compressions and rarefactions or sound waves. The frequency of the resultant sound wave is dependent on the thickness of the transducer element. The reverse is also true when the crystal is struck by a sound wave, it produces an electrical impulse.

Reviewing a diagram of the basic parts of a transducer shows the piezoelectric element with electrodes on either side. The electrodes are connected to an electrical source. Behind the piezoelectric element is a backing or damping material which is used to absorb any sound energy directed backward and to improve the shaping of the forward energy (Fig. 2.2).

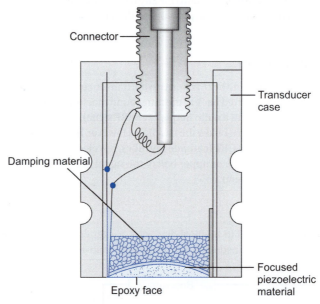

Fig. 2.2 Basic transducer construction

Beam Divergence

As the beam propagates it remains essentially parallel for a given distance. Then it begins to diverge. Where the beam begins to diverge is called the *far field*. Obviously it is better to examine objects in the *near field* because the beam there is parallel and reflecting surfaces tend to be more perpendicular, therefore, the returning information is of greater intensity. Many interfaces can also be detected in the far field but it becomes progressively more difficult to define these, the farther one goes into the far field.

The length of the near field is a function of the radius of the transducer. To lengthen the near field, one would either decrease the wavelength or increase the size of the transducer. The amount of divergence in the far field can be changed by using a *focused* transducer.

3

Real-time Ultrasound

Real-time scanning, at first a curiosity among clinicians, quickly surpassed static B-scanning as the major ultrasonic imaging mode. This almost immediate acceptance came about because real-time scanning is more flexible, displays anatomical motion that is otherwise undetected or confusing and offers images nearly as good as high-quality B-scanners.

In the hands of an experienced sonographer, real-time looks deceptively easy and quick. In fact real-time is fast but when handled improperly, fast can often mean missed information, poorly adjusted time-gain compensations (TGCs), inappropriate preprocessing, unused postprocessing and incomplete imaging data.

The sonographer must be able to adjust the machine according to the tissue presentations, scan all of the organs presented and provide a complete set of pictures for the attending physician. In other words, real-time shifts the skills emphasis from the sonographers transducer manipulations to correctly gathering the right images for a clinical conclusion.

Before picking up the transducer, the user must know what the exam is, what the clinical question is and why it was raised. Answers can be found on the exam request form, patient history and the results of previous tests and ultrasound exams.

Survey and Detail

The protocol has two parts—the survey and the specific scans for detailed imaging information.

The survey routine is the same for every patient, regardless of the final scanning sequence. Each survey begins with the use of a survey scan head, if one is available. These scan heads are usually medium-frequency, medium-focus transducers that penetrate the entire field of view and long focal zones.

The first observation is of the size and position, both internal and external, of the liver's left lobe. For a beginner, it is a good idea to mark the lower edge of the liver on the patients, skin with a water soluble pen with no scan-arm references to return to, the mark provides a good external reference.

The survey is continued by first moving to the patient's right. Always keeping parallel to the sagittal plane. This enables a regular view of organ size, the relationships among organs and the dynamics of each organ and great vessels. After surveying right, the operator returns to the midline and surveys left, again maintaining the scan plane parallel with the sagittal plane. The result is a collection of images that compose a complete survey of the upper abdomen from one point of view.

The next step is to change the scanning plane transversely to the sagittal plane and resurvey the upper abdomen. In these scans, the operator seeks details about the size of organs and vessels; angle of the boundaries; shape of organs and vessels; relationship among organs; positions of organs and boundaries relative to internal landmarks and to the external mark on the skin (patient breathing during the exam can displace organs and lesions).

The survey provides more than a calibration of organ size, shape and position, however, it offers a good mental three-dimensional image of the organs and their positions relative to one another, and sets the stage for the specific scans that follow.

Because scanning for specifics without landmarks can often yield disappointing results, the sonographer should have one or more internal references within an image. These references can include structures such as the aorta, the inferior vena cava, the superior mesenteric artery, the superior mesenteric vein, portal veins and the diaphragm.

The images should always have a common anatomical reference. For example, the patient's head or right hand side always appears on the image left.

In specific exams, following the upper abdominal survey, the pancreas is scanned first, before any breathing maneuvers introduce air into the stomach and gut. If air is already in the stomach, the gas may be displaced by having the patient drink a glass or two of water. This solution often gives a clear view of the pancreas. Water in the stomach often makes it easy to show the papilla of Vater and the common bile duct. Here real-time speed permits a thorough examination while the acoustical window is present.

The flexibility of the real-time scan head and image quality make studies of the gallbladder even more informative. A patient can be rolled while being scanned to observe the movement of gallstones or sludge. With this maneuver, a great deal can be learned about the condition of the bile simply by watching how fast things move in the gallbladder.

Showing all the bladder's border at 90° permits an accurate measurement of wall thickness; and the 90° position will minimize the beam-width artifacts that are common to most real-time systems.

The liver provides one of the best settings to view the changes in texture resulting from tumors. Here real-time adds a dimension not available to the B-scanner.

With real-time, it is possible to show the entire length of the renal artery and renal vein. These vessels should be included in every renal examination. Several views at 90° to the renal capsule can help differentiate between retro- and intraperitoneal masses. And real-time's flexibility enables the operator to stand the patient up to observe internal movements with leaning and tilting. The left kidney can be viewed through the spleen—a complete study requires imaging both kidneys.

Imaging vessels and the diaphragm through the spleen is easy but it requires following imaging conventions. Through the spleen is a view of the tail of the pancreas, which can sometimes be confused with food in the stomach. Real-time distinguishes the two because food in the stomach will move while the pancreatic tail is more stable.

When to Use Real-time

Whether or not to use a real-time system for a particular application depends on following factors:
1. Scanning field design, which may be linear or sector
2. Within the scan converter and
3. Frame rate.

The first deciding factor for a particular application is the pattern of the scanning field. For example, linear arrays produce a rectangular field in contrast to the pie-shaped fields of the sector scanner.

On the other hand, the sector scanner does not produce a uniform field. As a result, without special signal processing, the sector portion close to the transducer may be so badly overwritten that near imaging can be difficult or, in some cases, impossible.

A special need in obstetrical scanning is to gain a view of the fetal head in order to measure the biparietal diameter. The linear array is one of the best ways to deal with this imaging problem, a clinically well-accepted solution for this particular application.

On the other end of the spectrum, echocardiography uses sector scanners almost exclusively. Despite some successful applications of the linear array to echocardiography, it has not gained general acceptance within the cardiology community.

In addition, sector scanners are used more often than linear arrays for upper abdominal scanning. The narrow field in sector scanners close to the transducer provides an opportunity to circumvent some of the upper abdominal scanning problems, such as bowel gas and ribs. In general, linear arrays offer similar imaging capabilities but may not be able to explore some of the tighter spots as well as the sector scanner.

The second deciding factor for real-time applications is the size of the scanning head. Large sector scan heads, for example, have limited use in echocardiography but are useful in abdominal and obstetric scanning. Also large linear arrays will have limited use in standard abdomens but can be utilized in obstetric examinations.

Upper abdominal scanning and obstetrical scanning often rely on an ability to visually discriminate among signals coming from subtle lesions. At least 32 gray levels enable real-time scanning to depict and discriminate among subtle tissue difference. As a result, the real-time echocardiograph can use 16 or even fewer gray levels successfully, although the current trend is toward 64 gray levels.

Any real-time sonograph is limited, of course, by the line density in each scanning frame, the depth of display and the frame rate, in a combination that fits within very specific limits. Real-time systems with high line densities used for detailed abdominal scanning are not useful in echocardiography, because the high line density produces a frame rate too low to visualize a moving heart.

The contemporary real-time sonograph makes it possible to conduct a fast and effective exam. The automatic movement of the transducer beam, and the small size and light weight of the scan head provide freedom to move the transducer and the beam into new locations within the body. With the freedom to move comes the risk of moving improperly, which can result in loss of information and anatomical references that would normally be found with a B-scanner.

4

Introduction to Abdominal Scanning

Diagnostic ultrasound provides a unique method of examining structures beneath the skin surface. The image produced is cross-sectional, and sonography has a primary advantage over radiography by nature of its capacity to distinguish interfaces between soft tissue structures of the body. This ability plus the noninvasive and nontraumatic qualities of ultrasonography have resulted in ever increasing interest and use during recent years.

The next important step is to recognize an adequate scan, and how to achieve the same. In B-scanning the strongest echoes are produced when the sound beam is at right angles to an interface. For this reason it is often necessary to employ a compound sector scanning motion to record a maximum number of interfaces at perpendicularity.

Because the transducer spends approximately 99% of its time listening and less than 1% of its time sending the signal, it is important to develop a proper scanning speed so that every echo will be recorded. Scanning too fast results in many echoes being unrecorded. Scanning too slow allows the beam to concentrate too long on one particular area causing artifactual echoes to appear (Fig. 4.1).

The skin over the area of interest should be liberally coated with mineral oil or other suitable couplet to eliminate any air molecules between the transducer and the skin, thus providing maximum contact.

It is advisable to carry out scanning in an orderly fashion and to identify the anatomical position where transverse and longitudinal cross sections are taken by recording a preselected landmark. Most commonly used landmarks are:

- Umbilicus
- Xiphoid process
- Iliac crest
- Symphysis pubis.

Osseous structures are preferable because they do not change position.

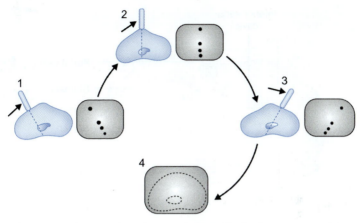

Fig. 4.1 As the transducer is moved across the body, an image of the body section transversed is built up on the storage screen

All recorded scans should be labeled for future reference with the following information:
- Patient's name
- Date
- Anatomical position
- Gain setting (whenever applicable).

The criteria for an adequate scan as described by Filly and Freimanis is helpful to the novice in evaluating a scan (Figs 4.2 and 4.3):
- Longitudinal scans
  - Well-defined anterior/posterior aortic walls on left side
  - Well-defined liver-diaphragm interface on right side.
- Transverse scans
  - Posterior liver surface well outlined
  - Anterior surface of spine seen
  - Adequate delineation of aorta and whenever possible the inferior vena cava
  - Adequate delineation of the left side of the spine on transverse scans.

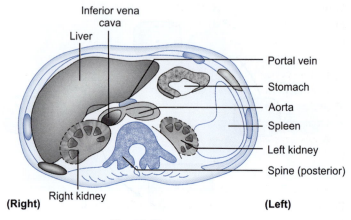

Fig. 4.2 Transverse, supine

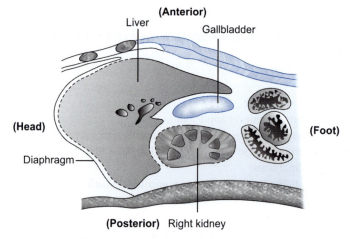

Fig. 4.3 Longitudinal, supine, 6 cm right

Examination Protocol

- Greet the patient
- Take the patients history (in a private place)
- Explain the procedure to the patient
- Instruct the patient on how to gown

- Complete 'paper work' while patient changes
- Review available clinical information
- Position patient on exam table:
  - As far to the edge of the table (near you) as possible
  - Elevate patients head as needed
  - Instruct patient to elevate arms if abdominal/kidney scans are being performed
  - Drape the patient
  - Apply appropriate contact-media.
- Set instrumentation/film devices, etc.
- Perform scans and record
  - Longitudinal, transverse and oblique if necessary
- Prepare and process films at completion of examination
- Release patient.

5

CHAPTER

Sonography of Soft Tissues

The soft tissues are a heterogeneous organ comprising the muscles, tendons, subcutaneous fat, fascia and skin.

Soft Tissue Abnormalities

- Mineralization
- Foreign bodies
- Trauma
- Infection
- Neoplasm
- Miscellaneous.

Mineralization

Abnormal soft tissue mineralization reflects in calcification or ossification. Calcification is defined as deposition of calcium in the normal or damaged tissues due to either disturbance in calcium or phosphorus-metabolism or due to tissue dystrophy.

The ossification is defined as calcification organized into trabeculae and cortex.

On ultrasound, calcification usually appears hyperechoic and shows posterior acoustic shadowing.

Foreign Bodies

All metal fragments except aluminum are radiopaque. All glass including ordinary machine glass which does not contain lead is radiopaque. Wood is not easily visible radiographically.

Ultrasound should be used for objects known to be nonradiopaque but not found on exploration.

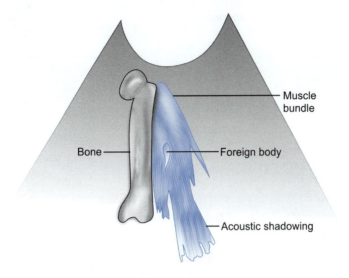

Fig. 5.1 Foreign body in soft tissue

Ultrasound shows a foreign body usually as an echogenic structure with posterior shadowing and has been found useful in the extremities and in the superficial soft tissues (Fig. 5.1).

Trauma

Trauma to muscle and tendon is reasonably common.

Ultrasound is most effective modality for evaluation of superficial tendons and muscles. Using a 7.5–10 MHz linear transducer most tendons and muscles can be evaluated properly.

Infection

Infection includes cellulitis, myositis, tendosinovitis and wound infection.

Ultrasound is sensitive to abnormalities and may characterize abscess.

Tendosinovitis: Ultrasound shows soft tissue swelling. Anechoic collection in the joint is displacement of pad of fat by anechoic collection.

Osteomylitis: Ultrasound may show marked cortical irregularity with abscess collection adjacent to bone. Under normal circumstances, there is no fluid collection adjacent to bone. If anechoic or hypoechoic collection are apparent

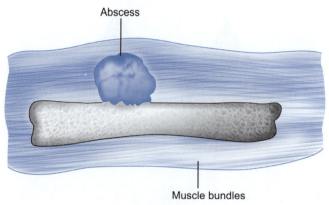

Fig. 5.2 Osteomylitis

adjacent to bone or within soft tissue infection should be suspected. The location of fluid with respect to bone is an important factor in differentiating acute osteomylitis from soft tissue abscess (Fig. 5.2).

Neoplasm

Ultrasound would be a good modality for evaluation of soft tissue neoplasm.

Ultrasound may show heterogeneous space occupying mass or lesion may show mixed echogenicity, calcification and shadowing, etc.

Miscellaneous

Muscles – Pathology of muscle can be well-defined by ultrasound and should be utilized as first imaging modality.

A 7.5 or 5 MHz transducer provides excellent results in two planes with good demonstration of sonographic palpation.

Ultrasound: A normal muscle appear as hypoechoic muscle bundle separating the hypoechoic lines as fibroadipose septa. The various muscle pathologies like muscle rupture, distraction of muscle fibers, abscess, hematoma, cyst and myositis ossificans can be well demonstrated.

6

Hepatic Sonography

Hepatic Ultrasound

Indications for Ultrasound

- To determine size, configuration, contour
- Ascites
- Jaundice
- Cystic disease
- Abscess
- Fever of unknown origin (FUO)
- Movement of diaphragm
- Primary carcinoma of liver
- Single defect, contour defect, or nonuniform uptake on isotope scan
- To localize lesion for liver biopsy.

Other Clinical Tests

- Liver function tests
  - Lab exams which are only screening procedures which if abnormal indicate some form of liver disease but do not indicate the specific disease
  - Alkaline phosphatase
  - Lactate dehydrogenase (LDH), serum glutamic-oxaloacetic trans-aminase (SGOT), serum glutamic pyruvic transaminase (SGPT)
  - Bilirubin (direct and indirect)
  - Fetal antigens
- Nuclear medicine
  - No hazard to patient
  - Cannot demonstrate lesion less than 2 cm
  - May be equivocal and is not specific for specific diseases

- Liver biopsy
  - Is of some hazard to patient although relatively painless
  - May miss lesion at biopsy (ultrasound may help accurately localize lesion)
- Physical exam
  - In obese patient or patient with ascites, may be difficult to palpate liver, to determine size and/or presence of irregularities
- Radiographic exam
  - Computerized axial tomography
  - Delivers radiation to patient
  - In some instances requires IV contrast agents to be administered
  - Permits visualization of anatomy in only one plane
  - Requires certain amount of intraorgan fat to provide good visualization.

Kidneys, Ureters and Bladder

Only will show liver edge and help determine size. Not of much value for liver size in patient with ascites.

Arteriography

Invasive procedure with certain degree of risk.

Cystic Lesions of Liver

- Congenital
  - Solitary-usually asymptomatic
  - Discovered only if large enough to be palpable
  - Polycystic-congenital anomalies of the bile ducts
  - 50% have polycystic kidneys
  - Liver disease usually causes no problem
  - Progressive renal failure
- Hemangioma
  - Lesion of blood vessels within the liver
  - Usually asymptomatic unless palpable
  - Rarely large ones can rupture
- Abscesses
  Location: Subphrenic—between liver and diaphragm
              Subhepatic—beneath liver
              Intrahepatic—within liver.

Types

- Bacterial
  - *Incidence and etiology:* 40% due to infection of organs drained by liver. About 10–15% occur with generalized sepsis.
  - *Symptoms and signs:* Persistent fever, sweats, chills, weight loss, nausea and vomiting, enlarged tender liver.
  - *Radiographic findings:* Decreased diaphragmatic movement. Basilar atelectasis, pneumonia, pleural effusion.
  - *Treatment:* Surgical drainage; antibiotics.
- Amebic
  - *Etiology:* Parasitic infection of large bowel.
  - *Symptoms:* Fever, sweats, weight loss, possibly tender enlarged liver.
  - *Location:* Usually single and most often in posterior portion of right lobe of liver.
  - *Radiographic findings:* Same as above.
  - *Treatment:* Same as above.

Primary Carcinoma of Liver

Types

- Liver cell (hepatoma).
- Bile duct cell (cholangioma).

Incidence

Only 1–2% of all malignancies 50–60 years old.

Increased incidence in patients with:

(1) Cirrhosis; (2) exposure to hepatotoxins.

Symptoms:	Right upper quadrant (RUQ) pain, ascites, tender mass
Diagnosis:	Must localize mass and do biopsy
Prognosis:	Usually die within 6 months
Treatment:	Resect if possible.

Metastatic Carcinoma to Liver

Incidence:	20 times more frequent than primary carcinoma. The 'double' blood supply of liver (from portal vein and from hepatic artery) makes it more susceptible to metastatic lesions.
Symptoms:	Usually referable to their primary carcinoma.

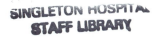

Diagnosis:	Palpable nodular liver; multiple defects on liver scan.
Treatment:	Treat primary tumor.
Cirrhosis:	Chronic diffuse liver disease with loss of cells.
Etiology:	Chronic alcoholism and poor nutrition, chronic hepatitis, etc.
	Rigid, small, firm, fibrotic liver with regenerating nodules.
Sequlae:	Portal hypertension—increased pressure in portal system due to increased resistance to flow through liver. Body attempts to compensate by developing numerous venous collaterals. Splenomegaly, GI hemorrhage, hemorrhoids, CNS problems.
	(*See* prominent venous channels on abdomen).
Cardiac cirrhosis:	Heart loses its ability to pump blood out so, lungs and liver become congested. Chronic congestion leads to cirrhotic changes in liver.
Jaundice:	*Extrahepatic obstruction:* Obstruction to flow of bile from liver by lesion outside of liver.
	For example: Stones in common bile duct, ampullary carcinoma, pancreatic carcinoma.
	Intrahepatic disease, for example, cirrhosis and hepatitis may also lead to jaundice.
Diaphragm movement:	Decreased motion of diaphragm with irritation of diaphragm or with phrenic nerve paralysis.

Examination of Liver

Size, Shape

Ultrasound can provide an excellent image of size, shape and configuration of liver.

Ascites

Another common request for liver examination is to rule out the presence of ascites. Quite often in patients who were thought to possibly have ascites were in fact suffering from excessive distension. So much so that even on ultrasound, the only portion of the liver visible was a small portion of the tail of the right lobe. Distension was so great that the liver substance was elevated up by gas filled bowel completely under the rib cage. Make an investigative midline scan of the pelvic region to check for a distended urinary bladder.

Because the cause of 'distension' and liver compression extremely high under the ribs was caused by a totally unsuspected pelvic mass. The expanding mass caused the displacement of bowel, and pressure on all adjacent structures including the liver occurs, presenting the previously described situation.

If, on the other hand, the patient does have ascites, the ultrasonic image can be extremely informative with regard not only to the presence of the ascites but to the severity or amount present. Ascites has been defined as an abnormal accumulation of serous fluid in the peritoneal cavity caused by increased venous pressure or a decrease of plasma albumin. The clear, yellowish fluid will coagulate when left to stand, but even in the body it may become turbid and contain blood or tissue debris. Ascites is most often associated with cardiac or renal deficiencies or cirrhosis of the liver.

It is interesting to note that in the earliest stages of ascites, when the volume of fluid is quite small, it often collects in the area between the liver and the right kidney, called Morrison's pouch, appearing as a thin, echo-free ribbon of fluid between the ultrasonically speckled-gray of the liver and the slightly homogeneous pattern of the kidney. As the amount of fluid builds, it begins to collect in the flank areas and appears as an echo-free zone between the abdominal wall and the liver and other organs. If the collection of fluid becomes massive, the echo pattern may reveal the liver and gallbladder compressed toward the center of the abdomen and frequently visually blocked by floating loops of black echo producing bowel.

If dietary therapy or diuretic measures fail to accomplish adequate relief from ascites, paracentesis must be performed. This procedure consists of tapping the abdominal fluid by introducing a hollow needle or trocar into the abdomen and draining off the excess fluid, which may exist in ranges of 1,000 cc's or more. If ever in doubt as to whether a homogeneous fluid collection is free or encysted, it is helpful to turn the patient to another position to see if the 'Fluid' will shift to the new dependent portion of the body, thereby changing contour as it is accommodated in this new area. Encysted fluid will not behave in this fashion as the thin walls of a cyst will maintain a more constant configuration and will not be free to drain into another area.

Jaundice

Another common reason for ultrasonic referral is the patient who is jaundiced. As mentioned previously, jaundice is the excessive accumulation of bile pigments and is evidenced by yellowing of the skin and the normally white sclera of the eyes.

The role of ultrasound in the jaundiced patient is to aid in determining whether the jaundice is medical or surgical in nature. Medical jaundice is the type caused by hepatocellular disease, while surgical jaundice is a result of obstruction. The area of obstruction is frequently due to a stone in the biliary system or pressure from an adjacent mass of the liver, to the gallbladder and from the gallbladder to the duodenum and out of the body. Both ascites and jaundice are frequently found in cirrhotic patients, a good example of medical jaundice caused by a hepatocellular disease.

Diaphragmatic Excursion

A very simple ultrasonic exercise that can be of value is determining the amount of movement of the diaphragm.

Decreased diaphragmatic movement is associated with irritation of the diaphragm or phrenic nerve paralysis. The ultrasonic technique for recording the excursion rate of the diaphragm is simple and takes less than 60 seconds to perform in most cases. A right longitudinal scan of the liver is obtained at approximately 4–8 cm right of the midline, with the patient in suspended inspiration. This image is left on the screen and a second scan is performed and superimposed over it while the patient is in a state of complete expiration. In the area of the diaphragm two, strong diaphragmatic, border echoes should be seen in a 'Normal' patient. Centimeter markers can be superimposed through this area and the actual amount of diaphragmatic excursion measured and recorded. Obviously, this technique is not always feasible on the left side of the abdomen unless a large left liver lobe, enlarged spleen or cardiac silhouette are present to provide a sonic window permitting recording and identification of the diaphragm.

Fever of Unknown Origin

Other more challenging reasons for evaluation are the existence of a palpable liver mass and investigation of the patient with persistent fever of unknown origin (FUO).

In outlining liver pathology, we are often confused because so many solid liver masses can have extremely homogeneous characteristics. Again, correlation of other diagnostic tests, particularly laboratory liver function tests can start us along the right investigative tracks.

Not only is ultrasound useful in outlining liver lesions, it can be used accurately to select the biopsy site of liver lesions thus, ensuring that the best possible area of the liver, the lesion itself, has been sampled. In patients, who present with fever of unknown origin, ultrasound can be used to rule out the presence of any infections process.

Liver Cysts

Congenital

The term 'congenital' means existing at birth. The congenital, benign solitary cyst of the liver is the most common primary cystic disease of the liver, and can be divided into two categories:

True cysts which are formed with an epithelial cell lining or false cysts which are lined by fibrous tissue. Most often these cysts are unilocular, although some have been described to contain separations. Usually they are small and discovered only incidentally during routine physical examinations. When they are large they may contain as much as a thousand cc's of fluid and eventually will cause the patient to complain of pressure-related pain.

The diagnostic pitfalls associated with solitary cysts of the liver are that they actually may be renal or adrenal in origin and mistakenly labeled as 'liver' cyst or that they may be echinococcal cysts (Figs 6.1 and 6.2), in which case puncture should be avoided. Follow-up studies of the cyst may be ordered and it is well to note that congenital cysts will show an echo-pattern change only if there has been hemorrhage within the cyst, while echinococcal cysts which may grow larger will also show changes in echo pattern. On rare occasions, a solitary cyst has been confused with the gallbladder.

Polycystic Disease of the Liver

Approximately 20–50% of patients with polycystic kidney disease (PKD) will also present with polycystic disease of the liver. This embryologically

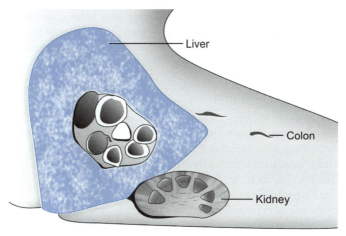

Fig. 6.1 Hydatid cysts (Longitudinal section)

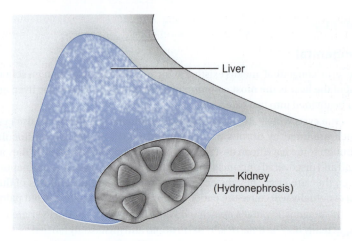

Fig. 6.2 Hydronephrosis simulating a hydatid (Longitudinal section)

determined condition can also coexist in the pancreas, spleen or lung. The typical echo pattern is of scattered, random-sized cystic structures throughout the liver parenchyma. The typical well outlined, echo-free structure is seen, and in addition the right kidney is also usually seen to be involved during the routine liver exam. It is an accepted technique to extend the limits of the liver exam, whenever polycystic disease is suspected to include a thorough investigation of the kidneys. Similarly, whenever kidneys are being evaluated and polycystic disease suspected, the liver of that patient should also be evaluated.

While both the liver and pancreas may develop lesions, death usually results because the lesions in the kidney eventually cause renal failure. It is important to remember that in adult polycystic disease, the condition is most apparent during the 40–50 years of life.

Acquired Cysts (Simple)

Acquired cysts are usually related to some types of trauma and actually from a pathologic point of view would be called false cysts because their walls are lined with fibrous tissue rather than the usual epithelial cells material. One of the most frequently found cysts of this type is the hydatid or echinococcal cyst. The liver seems to be the favored site, particularly the right posterior lobe. This is probably as a result of the excellent drainage of the intestinal area by the portal venous system. These cysts may grow unnoticed for years and may reach extremely large proportions of 15–20 cm in diameter before being discovered by palpation during physical exam. An interesting feature of this main cyst is its ability to develop 'daughter' cysts in large numbers and of varying sizes. Only over a period of many years when calcification deposits can be observed within the inner walls of these cysts would they be diagnostically accessible to X-rays. Ultrasonically this lesion usually appears as a very obvious homogeneous interruption of liver pattern. During its early stage, the mother cyst is very well visualized as well bordered and echo-free, but as the mother cyst fills with daughter cysts over an extended time period its liquid-like pattern changes. The appearance of multiple separations may cause confusion with polycystic liver disease. Usually if the patient is asymptomatic the cysts seen are most likely congenital. If the cysts are generally painful they are more likely to be acquired. Laboratory test can be extremely helpful in reaching a positive diagnosis. Obviously one extremely important fact to remember is that the echinococcal cyst should not be aspirated.

Abscesses

Abscesses are localized collections of pus which may be found anywhere in the body. They are named according to location and can be divided into two main groups—bacterial and amoebic.

Before collecting and settling in one spot the material that comprises the abscess is both liquid and solid. Once the collection in one location is established and necrosis begins, the abscess becomes more homogeneous looking, with only random areas of low level echo reflection coming from floating tissue debris. Most often the walls of an abscess appear shaggy and irregular but during the necrotic stage and depending on the type of surrounding body material they can develop more well-defined borders and be easily confused with cystic lesions. Once again attention to the patient's history regarding symptoms of infection, i.e. pain, fever, elevated WBC's, etc. will guide your thinking.

In discussing liver abscesses, we should turn our attention to the following locations:

Subphrenic—between liver and diaphragm (Fig. 6.3)

Subhepatic—beneath the liver

Intrahepatic—within the liver (Fig. 6.4).

At least 40% of the abscesses related to the liver will be the result of infection of some other organ that is drained by the liver. Other causes which have been named are penetrating ulcers, rupture of the gallbladder or extension from other abscesses such as parapelvic or appendiceal abscesses. Infection due to trauma has been reported as very rare. The treatment indicated is usually surgical drainage and or antibiotic therapy.

Because liver abscess can be multiple and small as well as large collections of fluid, it is extremely important that the entire liver be carefully examined.

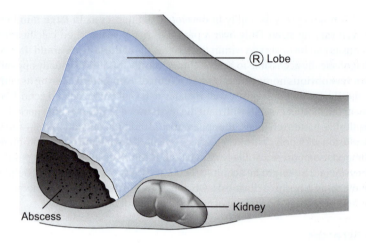

Fig. 6.3 Subphrenic abscess

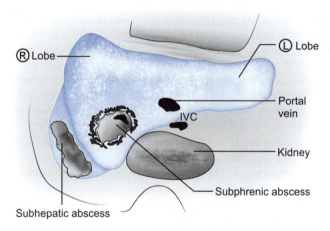

Fig. 6.4 Subphrenic and intrahepatic abscess (Transverse section)

Failure to direct the sound beam adequately up under the costal margin during longitudinal scans will result in incomplete imaging of the dome of the liver, a primary area of investigation for subphrenic collections. Extending the evaluation of the liver as far to the patient's right side will permit visualization of the hepatorenal angle or Morrison's pouch. This potential space is not only a good drainage area for ascitic fluid but for abscess formation.

One should repeat tests on the patient to chart the effectiveness of the drug program. Amoebic abscesses are most commonly seen in the middle age group and interestingly occur in males about four times more often than in females. The primary cause is from a parasitic infection of the bowel and the symptoms are of an enlarged and tender liver, sweating and possible weight loss. The parasites are communicated from man to man by way of fecally contaminated food or water. The conditions may be accompanied by dysentery in approximately half of the patient population. The amoebic hepatitis and eventually amoebic abscess. Ultrasonically, the abscess may or may not have well-defined borders relative to its size and the areas of necrosis associated with it. Lesions of long standing develop liquid centers filled with floating debris and are fond of locating in the dome of the liver or near the hepatic flexure of the colon.

Be cautious when examining for this mass and remember to use gain settings or transducers guaranteed to provide total penetration and reflection from the deepest most inaccessible areas of the liver. In former times, when less sophisticated equipment was all that was available, it was a routine procedure to perform several extremely high gain studies of the deepest aspects of the liver. Not infrequently, only this approach yielded the classical pattern of liver abscess. If even with today's improved equipment, you are faced with a large patient or one whose liver is primarily covered by ribs, this old 'trick' may still be invaluable.

Tumors

Benign

Any tumor which originates in the liver can generally be called a hepatoma.

We will discuss on hamartomas, adenomas and hemangiomas. The hemartoma can often be found in the liver in a variety of shapes and sizes ranging from less than a millimeter to more than 9 cm in size. The smallest hemartoma are actually composed of excessive and irregular bile ducts. When small, these lesions are generally round and smooth, but as they grow they become irregularly shaped, lobulated, capable of bulging out of the liver capsule and developing a stalk or pedicle. Usually they contain more fat than the surrounding liver tissue or parenchyma, but as they grow they cause some degree of atrophy in adjacent liver cells and may present an image that can be diagnostically confused with a focal area of cirrhosis. These nodules do not attain specific clinical significance until they reach such large proportions that they are noticeably space-occupying and can be palpated on physical exams. Their sonic pattern can be either more or less homogeneous than the surrounding liver tissue. The hemangioma on the other hand is a tumor

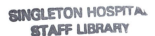

of the blood vessels of the liver and is generally seen as less echo producing structure when compared with the soft monotonous gray pattern of the liver. Small hemangiomas may appear during pregnancy but usually disappear afterwards.

Hepatic adenomas have been gaining most of the spotlight lately in discussions of benign liver tumors. Their gross appearance is quite similar to the hemangioma but recently they have been uncharacteristically associated with an unusually young patient group—young females who have been long time users of oral contraceptives. In this patient group, the tumor has occasionally reached such proportions that it has ruptured, causing sudden, severe internal hemorrhage and in some instances death. The growth of this lesion undergoes resolution when the oral contraceptive agents are discontinued.

Liver Tumors

Malignant

Primary carcinoma of the liver can be discussed in two major categories:
1. Carcinoma of the liver cell or hepatoma and
2. Carcinoma of the bile duct cell or cholangioma.

The incidence of primary liver cancer is actually small.

Only 1–2% of all liver malignancies are a primary type. It is generally associated with patients in the 50–60 year age group and shows an increased incidence in patients with cirrhosis or those who give a history of excessive exposure to hepatotoxins.

The symptoms are generally of right upper quadrant (RUQ) pain, a tender mass and ascites. In order to reach a diagnosis it is usually necessary to localize the mass and then biopsy it. The prognosis of a patient with primary carcinoma of the liver is not good, usually they die within 6 months. If possible resection of the tumor from the liver is the accepted method of treatment.

Interestingly, this lesion also appears far more often in males than in females and is given the dubious distinction of being the most frequent type of primary cancer in children up to 2 years of age, where it is apparently congenital.

Grossly, this mass usually appears as a massive nodule occupying the right lobe and frequently actually replacing it. While it is substantially solid, it may also contain areas of hemorrhage and necrosis which would yield a mixed echo pattern. It is possible for smaller 'daughter nodules' to be found scattered irregularly throughout the liver.

Primary carcinoma of the liver is a very confusing entity and may be accompanied by cirrhosis. As mentioned jaundice and ascites may develop or be accentuated as well as the patient's observation of a sudden enlargement of the abdomen. The laboratory tests of such a patient may demonstrate an increase in alkaline phosphatase and in 50% of the patients, the presence of fetal antigens. Primary carcinoma is then generally divided into three architectural categories:

1. Massive
2. Nodular and
3. Diffuse (the type most associated with cirrhotic changes).

Ultrasonic echo patterns that are specifically associated with primary carcinoma of the liver do not yet exist. Frequently, a well-defined heterogeneous solid lesion may be observed. Other times a 'bulls eye' pattern may be observed wherein a dense central echo producing structure surround by a ring or halo of less echo activity is seen. Confusion exists since each of these same descriptions also apply to metastatic lesions. The problem is even more accentuated if the patient also has cirrhosis.

In summary, the echo patterns that may be seen in primary liver carcinoma may be:

i. Increasingly echogenic
ii. Decreasingly echogenic
iii. Or a combination of the two; a mixed pattern.

In some patients, radio and chemotherapy may be indicated. In such patients, ultrasound can provide invaluable information concerning the response of the tumor to treatment.

Metastatic Tumors

The incidence of the metastatic cancer of the liver is approximately 20 times more frequent than primary carcinoma. The double blood supply of the liver from the portal vein and the hepatic artery makes this organ more susceptible to metastatic lesions.

The patient's symptoms are usually referable to their primary carcinoma. The patient may yield the impression of a palpably nodular liver on physical exams and multiple defects on nuclear liver scan. The treatment indicated is to find and treat the primary tumor, to stop-once and for all, its metastatic involvement of the liver. The actual picture of this condition varies widely from the presence of only a few small-to-moderately sized nodules. They change the appearance of the edge of the liver (where they tend to group) from being smooth to lumpy. The more numerous and closely spaced, the nodules are the more irregular the liver feels and appears on ultrasound. Because these lesions tend to become vascularly inadequate the larger nodules are subject to degeneration or necrosis and thus, can present a mixed echo pattern.

In patients with moderate to severe nodular involvement, the ultrasonic characteristic are loss of smooth and regular liver outline and the production of very irregular liver border reflections. Symptoms may include hepatic enlargement, pain, distention of the abdomen, fever, anemia and malaise (or the blahs). When sufficient liver involvement exists, the patient may become jaundiced as a result of the obstruction of extrahepatic biliary ducts. The only significant liver lab test is the presence of bromsulphalein and moderate serum alkaline phosphatase.

Hepatocellular Disease

The two major hepatocellular diseases we will discuss are cirrhosis and hepatitis.

Cirrhosis is a chronic diffuse liver disease resulting in the loss of functioning liver cells. There are varying types of cirrhosis which is marked by the atrophy or shriveling of the organ. Chronic retention of bile can cause biliary cirrhosis. Fatty infiltrating cirrhosis occurs when fat invades the liver cells and Laennec's cirrhosis refers to a specific fibrotic replacement of liver cells.

The clinical picture of the patient's cirrhosis will vary depending upon which form of the disease exists. The causes or etiology of cirrhosis that are most common are:

1. Chronic alcoholism and poor nutrition.
2. Chronic hepatitis.

The clinical picture, particularly in the more extreme cases, is very visibly dramatic. In the patient with biliary cirrhosis it is common to find elevated temperature and WBCs. In all cases, poor to severe liver function is seen. Most likely this is due to the extreme change in circulation which is present in cirrhotic patients. Normally the portal vein carries food-rich blood from the intestinal tract to the liver for processing. When the parenchymal cells of the liver are normal this activity is carried out with ease and rapidity. When however, liver cells become inflamed or infiltrated by fat or fibrous connective tissue, the hard working portal venous system begins to back up with large amounts of blood, it has not been able to direct into and through the liver. The venous system is extremely capable of distending to hold unusually large amounts of blood for short periods of time but not indefinitely. The body, presented with this logistics problem, attempts to compensate for the overload by shunting the excess blood into other adjacent venous channels. The situation known as portal hypertension usually first seen as excess blood being diverted to smaller caliber vessels such as those lining the esophagus. Without relief of this problem these overly stressed smaller vessels may rupture. In the esophagus this condition is referred to as esophageal varices and the blood can be found in the form of thick, black tarry stools or if severe bleeding occurs the patient may present with 'coffee ground' emesis so-called because of the emesis of blood which has been acted upon by stomach secretions until it does indeed resemble a dark brown, granular appearing substance. Dilatation of the abdominal veins may occur to such an extent that they are visibly present as thickened, rope-like channels disrupting the normally smooth appearance of the abdominal wall. Smaller, capillary ruptures are commonly seen particularly in the superficial vessels of the nose and cheeks, causing a reddish-purple discoloration from multiple fine ruptured capillaries. Palmar erythema or a reddening of the palms of the patient's hands may occur. Eventually the patient suffers from anemia, splenomegaly and bone marrow changes. Ascites, jaundice, psychic disturbances (notably delirium tremers or the 'DT'S') occur. In the early stages of portal hypertension, the liver may become swollen with congested blood. In the end stages, the liver has generally shrunken and hardened yet the painfully thin patient presents with a grossly swollen abdomen because of ascites.

In most extreme cases of alcoholic cirrhosis, the patients are also suffering from varying degrees of malnutrition thus, preventing the liver from calling on its marvelous restorative owners to reverse the tide of the disease. The ultrasound echo pattern of the cirrhotic patient is the replacement of the almost monotonously boring gray, low level echoes reflected from normal liver parenchyma to uncharacteristically large numbers of high density echo reflections. In the alcoholic patient, we tend to see two separate patterns. The patient with early alcoholic cirrhosis presents with an enlarged increasingly echogenic liver and some degree of portal hypertension, induced by dilated portal vessels covering the liver. In the advanced patients, because of progressive fibrosis the liver may appear large or small but will contain sufficient collections of fibrous material, so as to be markedly sound attenuating. Small hepatic venous structures will be obliterated and the portal system become irregularly shaped and run a tortuous course. The splenic vein may also become markedly dilated and an increase in splenic size also may be noted.

A possible diagnostic pitfall exists when regenerating areas or nodules of cirrhotic liver are mistaken for other mass lesions. Once again high-lighting the importance of clinical correlation. Cardiac cirrhosis, a condition which causes the heart to lose its ability to pump blood out, so that both the lungs and liver become congested. This chronic congestion may lead to cirrhotic changes in the liver. Another diagnostic pitfall in such a patient may be the confusion of a pleural effusion for ascites. Pleural effusions collect in the posterior aspects of the lung and would, therefore, appear as supradiaphragmatic area of echolucency, unlike the typical ascitic pattern which appears in the abdominal cavity as an echolucency between or around the liver and the diaphragm.

Ultrasonic Anatomy of the Liver

Liver Size and Shape

The contour and shape of the liver are dependent on the size of the lateral segment of the left lobe and the length of the right lobe. In addition, both of these features affect our ability to demonstrate abdominal structures adjacent to the liver. The left lobe is always smaller than the right, but it varies considerably in size from individual to individual. It may be congenitally small or atrophic. The degree to which the left lobe (particularly its lateral segment) extends toward the left and its craniocaudal dimension are key features in ultrasonic visualization of the pancreatic region. The greater the size of the lateral segment of the left lobe, the more likely one is to clearly observe pancreatic tissue.

The body habitus of the patient may affect these parameters. In patients with large anteroposterior diameter, the liver usually extends only slightly to the left of the midline. When the left lobe of the liver is small and the anteroposterior diameter of the patient is great, the upper retroperitoneum and even the gallbladder are exposed to interposition of bowel. This greatly complicates the obtaining of high-quality images of the aorta, vena cava, celiac and mesenteric vessels, pancreas and gallbladder.

The length of the right lobe determines the clarity of images of the right kidney in the supine position. Additionally, the longer the right lobe, the less likely it is that bowel gas in the hepatic flexure of the colon will obscure ultrasonographic detail of the right upper quadrant. Riedel's lobe, more common in women, is a tongue-like projection of the right lobe that may extend to the iliac crest. On both ultrasound and nuclear medicine studies it is positioned relatively anteriorly. While Riedel's lobe is anteriorly positioned, it appears to represent an enlargement of both the anterior and posterior segments of the right hepatic lobe. Occasionally Riedel's lobe is clinically or radiologically mistaken for a pathologic lesion. However, an echogenic parenchymal pattern identical with that of the remainder of the liver assures normalcy on the ultrasonogram.

Portal and Hepatic Venous Anatomy

Because of its highly constant course and the relative ease of visualization by sonography, the intrahepatic portal venous system may be employed as a specific indicator of the position of the ultrasonographic tomographic plane through the liver. The main portal vein (MPV) approaches the portal

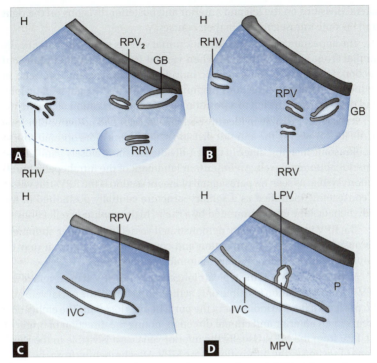

Figs 6.5A to D Diagrams of sequential sections through RPV and porta hepatis in frontal and longitudinal projections. Ultrasonograms (A to D) correspond to the planes of sections (A to D) in the diagrams
Abbreviations: H, head; RHV, right hepatic vein; GB, gallbladder; IVC, inferior vena cava; RRV, right renal vein; LPV, left portal vein; MPV, main portal vein; P, pancreas; RPV, right portal vein (A: angle of inclination at the origin of the LPV from the horizontal)

hepatis in a rightward, cephalic, and slightly posterior direction with the hepatoduodenal ligament. Near the porta hepatis it comes into contact with the anterior surface of the inferior vena cava (IVC). This important anatomic relationship specifically identifies the portal vein and, in addition, occurs at or very near the porta hepatis. Identification of the exact location of the porta hepatis is important in many clinical scanning situations. The point of contact of the portal vein with the IVC serves well as a general indicator of the location of the liver hilus (Figs 6.5A to D).

Entering the porta hepatis, the MPV divides into a smaller, more anterior, and more cranial left portal vein (LPV) and a larger, more posterior, and more caudal right portal vein (RPV). The portal veins then branch into medial and lateral divisions on the left and anterior and posterior divisions on the right and become intrasegmental in their courses.

The appearance of the intrahepatic portal venous system is dramatically similar from patient to patient when viewed from parasagittal planes of section. Displays the characteristic morphologic changes that are seen in sequential parasagittal sections beginning laterally in the right hepatic lobe and proceeding to the left to a position beyond the bifurcation of the MPV.

It is usually possible to identify both the anterior and posterior divisions of the RPV. However, the anterior division usually has a more optimal course for ultrasonic imaging, since in most individuals it more closely parallels the anterior abdominal wall. An important landmark of the intrahepatic portal venous system as seen on parasagittal planes of section is the RPV. This vessel is consistently identified as a solitary structure centrally positioned in the right hepatic lobe and surrounded by a rim of high-amplitude reflections.

The RPV is the most easily demonstrated vessel in the upper abdomen. Because of its ease of identification and consistent appearance, it may be employed with confidence as an anatomic reference point.

Also characteristic is the typical elongation of the MPV at the origin of the LPV. This configuration is visible only at the bifurcation of the portal vein and it represents a precise indicator of the porta hepatis location. The elongation occurs in an anterior and cranial direction, noting the direction of origin of the LPV from the MPV. Usually the inferior vena cava is visible in the same plane of section as the bifurcation of the MPV. After branching from the MPV, the LPV proceeds cranially along the anterior surface of the caudate lobe and then abruptly turns anteriorly. After giving off branches to the caudate lobe, it divides into medial and lateral second order portal branches supplying the segments of the left lobe.

On transverse sections, the intrahepatic portal system is also characteristic in appearance. Variation is found in the angle of entry of the RPV into the right hepatic lobe and, again, in the size and angle of origin of the LPV as its branches from the MPV. Most frequently the LPV originates from the MPV at a relatively shallow angle. Thus, the LPV is usually identified in a more cephalad location than the RPV.

The hepatic veins are usually divided into three major components. These are the right, middle and left hepatic veins. The right hepatic vein is always the largest, and the left hepatic vein is usually the smallest. The right hepatic vein enters the anterior or right anterior surface of the inferior vena cava. The left hepatic vein may enter the left anterior surface of the vena cava or may appear to enter directly into the right atrium. In many individuals, a long horizontally running branch of the right hepatic vein is identified coursing between the anterior and posterior divisions of the RPV (Fig. 6.6).

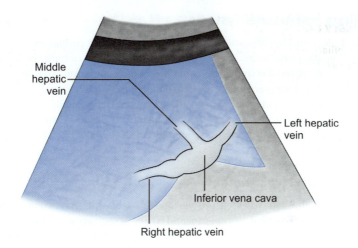

Fig. 6.6 Right, middle and left hepatic veins entering the right lateral, anterior and left lateral aspect of inferior vena cava (IVC)

Several features of the sonographic appearances of both portal and hepatic veins have been helpful in distinguishing between them. These distinguishing characteristics result from differences in the courses of hepatic and portal veins. Hepatic veins course between the hepatic lobes and segments, whereas the major portal branches course within the lobar segments. Hepatic veins drain toward the right atrium, whereas portal veins emanate from the porta hepatis. Thus, the diaphragm, a cranially situated structure, can serve as the reference point for recognition of hepatic veins, whereas the porta hepatis, more caudally located, is the anatomic reference point for portal veins.

Any large vein situated near the diaphragm may be considered a hepatic vein, conversely, any large venous structure situated near the porta hepatis may be considered a portal vein. An anatomic corollary of this feature dictates that the caliber of a hepatic venous radical becomes progressively greater the nearer, it courses toward the diaphragm, whereas the caliber of a portal venous radical is greater the nearer the vessel lies to the porta hepatis.

An additional feature is easily assessed, but it is less reliable in distinguishing the system of origin of an observed intrahepatic venous structure, the presence of high-amplitude reflections surrounding an intrahepatic venous radical suggests a portal venous origin, and the absence of such echoes suggests a hepatic venous origin.

Biliary and Arterial Systems

The biliary and hepatic arterial systems course in close contiguity with the intrahepatic portal veins. The extrahepatic components of both the biliary and hepatic arterial systems are visible within the hepatoduodenal ligament in a relatively large percentage of normal individuals. It is unusual to identify intrahepatic components of either of these systems. Occasionally, tiny tubular structures can be identified coursing adjacent to the RPV and less often the LPV. Undoubtedly these represent either intrahepatic biliary or arterial components.

Segmental Liver Anatomy

Essentially, the liver is divided into two lobes, each of which has two segments. The right lobe is divided into anterior and posterior segments, and the left lobe is divided into medial and lateral segments. The term quadrate lobe referred to a portion of the medial segment and the caudate lobe (Figs 6.7A and B).

The main lobar fissure divides the liver into its true anatomic right and left lobes. This fissure is found in a line joining the gallbladder fossa with the inferior vena cava. Both of these structures are easily seen on ultrasonograms, but determining the place of the line joining them is difficult. By contrast the middle hepatic vein, which is frequently identified, courses within the main lobar fissure. This vein divides the right lobe from the left lobe, but it can more appropriately be considered as dividing the anterior segment of the right lobe from the medial segment of the left lobe.

The right segmental fissure divides the anterior and posterior segments of the right lobe. The anterior and posterior divisions of the RPV course centrally in these segments. A long branch of the right hepatic vein, which is commonly observed on both transverse and longitudinal ultrasonograms courses within the right segmental fissure and bisects the anterior and posterior right portal divisions. This basic relationship allows a reasonably accurate ultrasonographic estimation of the positions of the anterior and posterior segments of the right lobe.

The left segmental fissure divides the left lobe into medial and lateral segments.

For ease of ultrasonic identification, the left intersegmental fissure can be conveniently considered as having cranial, middle and caudal thirds. The left hepatic vein courses within the cranial aspect of the left intersegmental fissure, thus dividing the cephalic portions of the medial and lateral segments of the hepatic lobe. The falciform ligament, a remnant of the fetal portion of the ventral mesentery extending between the LPV and the anterior abdominal wall, divides the caudal portions of the medial and lateral left hepatic segments.

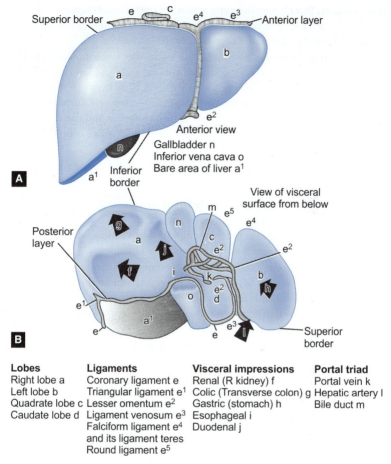

Figs 6.7A and B Digestive system—the liver

The falciform ligament is not commonly identified on ultrasonograms unless ascites is present or in patients who lack ascites, fibrofatty tissue is enclosed in the ligament. However, the ligamentum teres hepatis, which runs in the inferior or free edge of the falciform ligament, is frequently noted.

The middle third of the left intersegmental fissure can be identified by observing the course of the LPV. The LPV initially courses over the caudate lobe's anterior surface and generally toward the patient's left side. However, in this initial portion it does not give off branches to the lateral and medial segments. Before the segmental branches arise, the LPV makes an abrupt anterior turn. This change in course occurs in the left intersegmental fissure and can be employed as an indicator of the middle third of the fissure that divides the medial and lateral segments of the left lobe.

The caudate lobe must be considered separately, since it receives portal venous and hepatic arterial blood from both the right and left systems. The caudate lobe is the posterior portion of the liver lying between the fossa of the inferior vena cava and the fissure of the ligamentum venosum. The tissue lying between this fissure having ligamentum venosum and the caval fossa represents caudate lobe parenchyma. The caudate lobe lies cephalic to the bifurcation of the MPV.

Liver: Technique

Patient is in fast for minimum of 6 hours. Transducer should be 3.5 MHz frequency for adult. The overall gain should be set to display medium amplitude echoes in the liver parenchyma without producing artificial echoes in fluid filled structures such as portal vein or gallbladder.

Beginning with longitudinal sections, the transducer is placed at the costal margin and aimed as high as possible on the right hemidiaphragm, patient is requested to inspire deeply and to suspend respiration at end of inspiration. Linear motion is used to generate a longitudinal image using this technique complete volume of liver is scanned.

Transverse scans are obtained beginning at the immediate subxiphoid position, in suspended deep inspiration. The full liver cannot be visualized at one scan.

Because the liver lies under the costal margin, the most anterior portion of right and left lobes and most extreme lateral portion of right lobe of liver are frequently obscured by ribs.

Lateral aspect of right lobe of liver is best seen in right posterior oblique position; with the patient's right side down on scanning table and left side elevated. With the patient's right arm elevated above the head to help elevate the right ribs. Longitudinal and transverse scans can be obtained along the costal margin.

Anterior portions of right and left lobe of liver are best seen in transverse scan with patient in supine position. Scan is angled towards the head of the patient, again in deep inspiration.

Scans in transverse plane are best for evaluation of the left lobe, and oblique scans paralleling the right intercostal margin are best for the right lobe.

Ultrasound Appearances of Liver

Ascites

In early ascites, a thin layer of fluid occupies the hepatorenal angle. With increasing ascitis fluid starts collecting superior to liver and then inferior to liver. Gallbladder wall thickness may be seen (Figs 6.8 and 6.9).

Acute Hepatitis

There is moderate hepatomegaly. The attenuation will be normal. A transitory enlargement of pancreas is common and is considered an associated sign in acute pancreatitis (Fig. 6.10).

Chronic Hepatitis

It may be seen as increase in attenuation and appearance of micronodules (Fig. 6.11).

Cirrhosis

There is increased number of fine parenchymal echoes in a normal gain setting. There is poor penetration of beam because by increased absorption

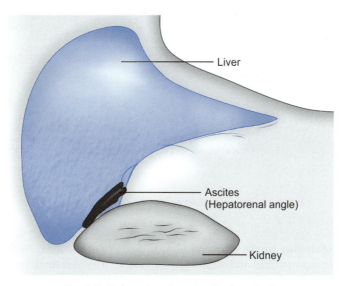

Fig. 6.8 Early ascites (Longitudinal section)

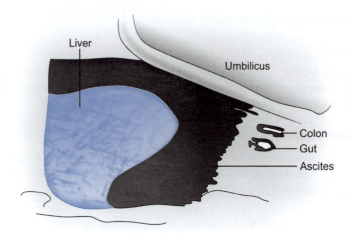

Fig. 6.9 Moderate ascites (Longitudinal section)

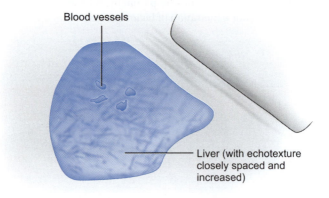

Fig. 6.10 Early alcoholic cirrhosis (Longitudinal section)

and scattering by the fatty and fibrotic changes of the liver. Sometime posterior part of liver and diaphragm may not be visualized. Ascitis may also develop behind the liver. Regenerating nodules in a cirrhotic liver may appear sonolucent with poorly defined borders (Fig. 6.12).

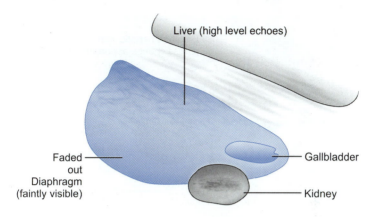

Fig. 6.11 Fatty changes (Longitudinal section)

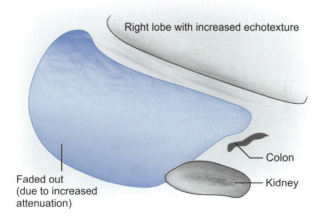

Fig. 6.12 Cirrhosis (Longitudinal section)

Portal Hypertension

Determining portal hypertension by ultrasound is usually easy. Dilatation of splenic vein-associated with splenomegaly is often seen. Dilatation of portal vein is easily visible. Varices are visible near the splenic hilum (Figs 6.13 to 6.15).

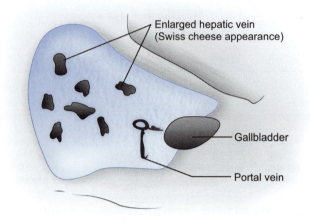

Fig. 6.13 Congestive heart failure (Longitudinal section)

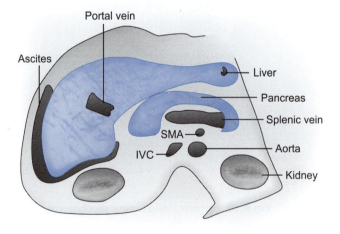

Fig. 6.14 Portal hypertension (Transverse section)

Solitary Liver Cyst

It displaces the smooth wall echo-free feature, together with characteristic distal enhancement (Fig. 6.16).

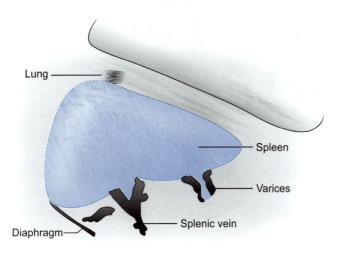

Fig. 6.15 Varices around the splenic vein (Longitudinal section)

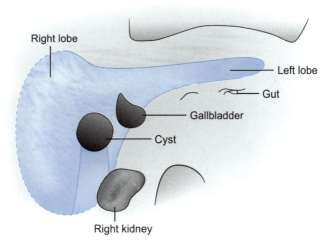

Fig. 6.16 Solitary liver cyst (Transverse section)

Polycystic Liver

Liver is enlarged. Large cysts show distal enhancement. Small cysts may not show clear band of echo enhancement (Fig. 6.17).

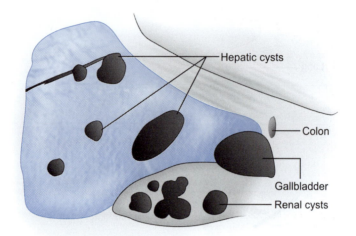

Fig. 6.17 Polycystic liver (Longitudinal section)

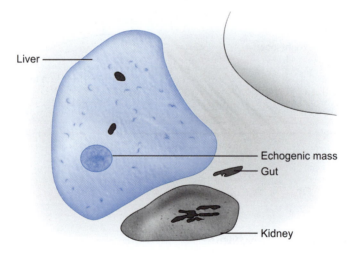

Fig. 6.18 Hemangioma (Longitudinal section)

Hemangioma

An echogenic lesion of different sizes may be seen in anywhere in liver parenchyma. These can be multiple (Figs 6.18 to 6.20).

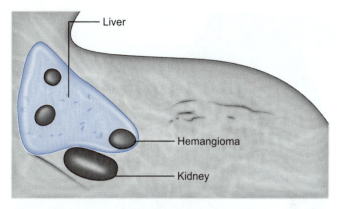

Fig. 6.19 Multiple hemangioma-neonates (Longitudinal section)

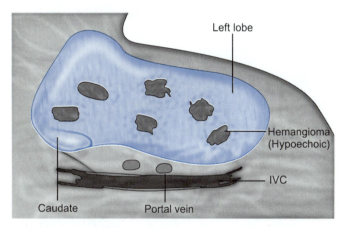

Fig. 6.20 Multiple hemangioma (Longitudinal section)

Cavernous Hemangioma

Echo-free focal lesion with an irregular or lobulated wall and absence of distal enhancement (Fig. 6.21).

Metastases

Focal deposit: It is a region of reduced reflectivity. The margins are usually ill-defined and its attenuation is the same as surrounding liver parenchyma.

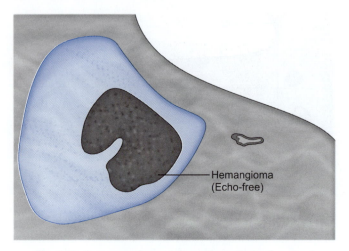

Fig. 6.21 Cavernous hemangioma (Longitudinal section)

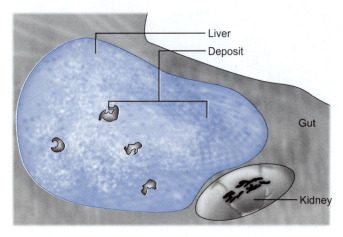

Fig. 6.22 Liver metastases (echo poor) (Longitudinal section)

Thus, they neither shadow nor produce distal enhancement and the echotexture is not noticeable distinct from that of the surrounding liver (Figs 6.22 to 6.24).

Differential diagnosis — Abscess
— Hemangioma
— Focal hepatitis (inacute alcoholic hepatitis).

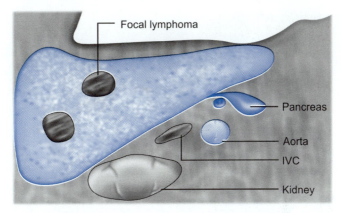

Fig. 6.23 Lymphoma focal (Transverse section)

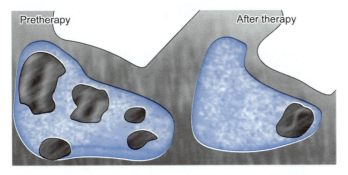

Fig. 6.24 Liver metastases (Improvements on therapy)

Echogenic Deposits

The margins are often ill-defined and these also neither shadow nor enhance. The increase reflection they produce probably correlate with increased vascularity and connective tissue content (Fig. 6.25).

    Differential diagnosis   — Ligamentum teres
                                    — Perinephric fat.

Bull's Eye Deposit

A central area of necrosis within a nodule will show as a sonolucent middle with an echo producing ring around it.

    Differential diagnosis   — Abscess.

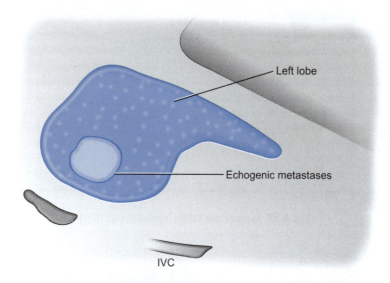

Fig. 6.25 Liver metastases—echogenic (Longitudinal section)

Calcific Deposits

Calcification in tumors show bands of shadowing beyond intensely echogenic foci (Fig. 6.26).

Cystic Deposits

Necrotic deposits contain fluid and show enhanced sound transmission. The fluid content shows some debris. The walls are irregular (Fig. 6.27).

> Differential diagnosis — Abscess
> — Simple cyst.

Generalized Involvement

• Mouth eaten—any tumor.
• Echo poor—lymphoreticular tumors.
• Fine texture—miliary metastases.

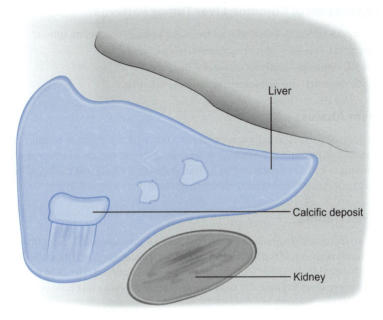

Fig. 6.26 Liver metastases—calcific deposit (Longitudinal section)

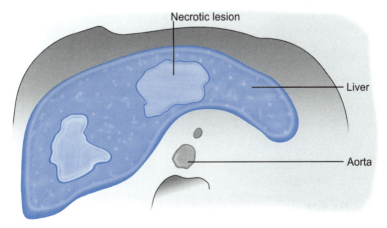

Fig. 6.27 Liver metastases—cystic (Transverse section)

Implication of Common Liver Tumor Patterns

Echo poor deposits—secondaries from any primary malignant tumor.
Echogenic deposits—gut or urogenital tract primary.
Calcific deposits—ovary or colorectal primary.
Cystic deposits—mucin secreting deposits sarcoma.

Liver Abscess

Hepatic abscess is usually a sonolucent mass with an irregular border. The number of internal echoes varies according to the nature of abscess and amount of cellular debris within it. The abscess may be single pocket of or it may be loculated, containing multiple pockets (Figs 6.28 to 6.31).

Liver Trauma

Liver trauma is indicated by ultrasound as a hematoma collection. A hematoma gives rise to a fluid band along the surface of organ. If the collection is subscapular, the peripheral margin will be well outlined. The fluid will not change position dramatically with a change in position as a free fluid or ascitis.

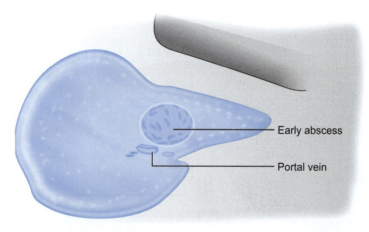

Fig. 6.28 Pyogenic liver abscess—early (Longitudinal section)

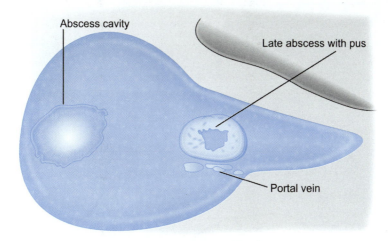

Fig. 6.29 Pyogenic liver abscess—late (Longitudinal section)

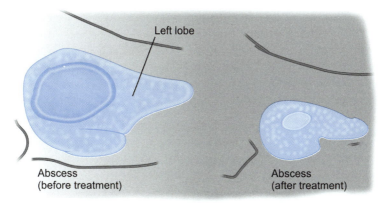

Fig. 6.30 Amebic abscess (response to therapy) (Longitudinal section)

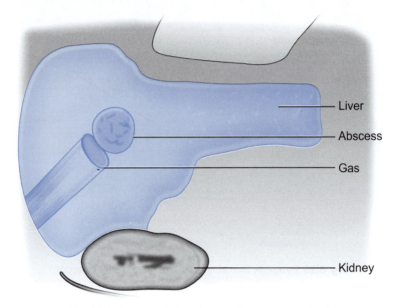

Fig. 6.31 Gas containing abscess (Transverse section)

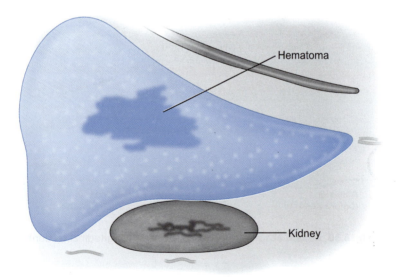

Fig. 6.32 Liver trauma (Longitudinal section)-I

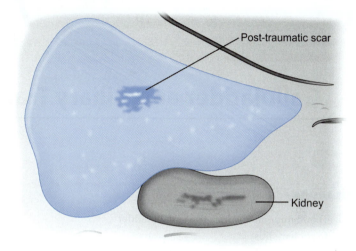

Fig. 6.33 Liver trauma (Longitudinal section)-II

Intrahepatic hematomas produce heterogeneous echoes with occasionally semisolid areas.

A fresh hematoma may appear mostly cystic, but with time and organization of blood it may take on a solid or mixed appearance. Nothing subtle changes in tissue texture may also be necessary in less obvious cases (Figs 6.32 and 6.33).

7

Gallbladder and Biliary Tract

Indications

- Size, configuration and location of gallbladder
- Acute cholecystitis
- Abscess
- Carcinoma of extrahepatic bile ducts
- Choledochal cysts
- Cholangiocarcinoma.

Anatomy

- It is located on inferior edge of liver between right and left lobes. Divisions—Fundus, body, infundibulum (Fig. 7.1). Gallbladder up to 10 cm long and 3–5 cm diameter
- Cystic duct 3 cm long
- Common bile duct 8 mm diameter and 2–3 cm long.

Physiology of the Gallbladder

Bile is constantly being secreted by the liver cells starting in the minute channels in the liver called bile canaliculi. From these small channels, they converge into the right and left hepatic ducts. These ducts drain into the main hepatic duct to form the common bile duct.

The common bile duct enters the duodenum at the site where it meets the pancreatic duct at the ampulla of Vater. When there is no food in the upper digestive tract, most of the bile is diverted into the gallbladder, where it is stored and concentrated by absorption of fluid. Following a meal, bile enters the small bowel due to relaxation of the sphincter of Oddi, contraction of the gallbladder, and increased bile secretion by the liver. This process is initiated by the enzyme cholecystokinin, which is released when fats and proteins

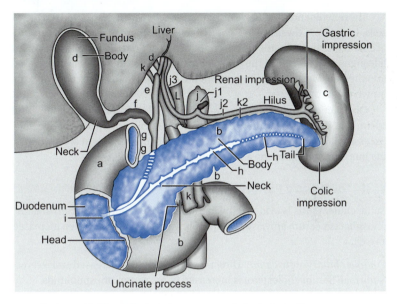

Fig. 7.1 Gallbladder

Right and left hepatic duct d
Common hepatic duct e
Cyst duct f
Common bile duct g
Duodenal papilla i
Abdominal aorta j
Celiac trunk j1

Splenic artery j2
Common hepatic j3
Superior mesenteric artery j4
Portal vein k
Superior mesenteric vein k1
Splenic vein k2
Inferior vena cava l

reach the duodenum. Bile plays an important role in the intestinal breakdown and absorption of fat and is the vehicle of excretion of the end product of hemoglobin breakdown.

The amount of bile excreted daily is about 250–1000 mL. Bile is made-up of mostly water, bile salts, and their organic substances in small amounts including cholesterol. Bile salts are derived from metabolism of hemoglobin. In addition to digesting and absorbing fats, bile also emulsifies fats into minute particles. This provides for greater surface area for pancreatic lipase to act upon the fats in further digestion. At the end of their digestive function, bile salts are returned by the portal system to the liver for reuse.

Cholesterol makes up a small part of the bile, but increased amounts tend to cause a higher incidence of gallstone formation. Addition of bile salts helps to keep cholesterol in solution to stimulate bile flow, and keep the concentration of cholesterol down.

The reticuloendothelial system contains cells which destroy old red blood cells. In the liver, these are the Kupffer cells. Bile pigment is the end product of the breakdown of hemoglobin contained in old red blood cells. The major bile pigment is bilirubin. The 0.5–2.0 g of bilirubin produced daily is secreted into the bile. Most of the bile pigment are excreted in the feces and impart a brown color to the feces.

Obstruction of a bile duct prevents flow of bile and the increase secretion by the liver causes a back flow of bile in the liver with obstruction to bile flow. Excessive fat is found in the feces due to lack of digestion and absorption in the intestine caused by the absence of bile salts.

Tests for Biliary Functions

Acute cholecystitis is evidence by increase in BSP retention, serum alkaline phosphatase, serum amylase and lipase are elevated. SGOT is often increased as well.

Complete biliary obstruction: Direct serum bilirubin is increased and indirect is normal. Serum cholesterol is increased as are serum phospholipids.

Obstruction of one hepatic bile duct: Serum bilirubin remains normal. Serum alkaline phosphatase is markedly increased.

Cancer of gallbladder and bile duct (3%).

The laboratory findings of associated duct obstruction are of progressively increasing severity.

The stool is often positive for occult blood. Anemia is also present.

Intermittent stones in bile duct cause fluctuating laboratory findings.

Radiographic Ways to Study Gallbladder

Oral cholecystogram: Ultrasound will not replace this but will be utilized if patient's gallbladder does not visualize or if patient is jaundiced.

Intravenous cholangiogram: It requires intravenous infusion of contrast. Hazardous in that reactions occur to contrast. If patient's bilirubin is highly elevated, chance of visualization of biliary system is less.

Percutaneous transhepatic cholangiography: It requires introduction of cannula into liver and cannulization of bile duct and injection of contrast. It is not without hazard but is safer now with newer methods.

Disease of Gallbladder

Stones: Different types of stones with cholesterol stones being most common type.

Incidence of calcification in gallstones = 20%

If calcification is seen on plain film of abdomen must prove that this is within the gallbladder rather than in kidney, lymph nodes or soft tissue. Do X-ray to view right lateral view of abdomen.

Acute cholecystitis: It occurs when stone impacts in the cystic duct.

Symptoms: Right upper quadrant pain, nausea and vomiting fever, elevated white blood cell count, pain radiates to shoulder. The remission of symptoms is 75%.

Chronic cholecystitis: Numerous episodes of acute cholecystitis.

Common duct stone: It occurs when stone migrates from gallbladder into common bile duct and obstructs that duct. Result is pain, jaundice, fever, chills.

Carcinoma of Gallbladder

Rare.

Congenital Anomalies of Gallbladder

Choledochal cysts: Localized cystic dilatation of common bile duct.

Symptoms: Occur during first 2 decades of life. The intermittent symptoms are occurring when cyst distends and compresses common bile duct causing jaundice, pain and a mass.

Treatment: Drain surgically into duodenum with good results.

Biliary Tree: Technique

Overnight fast is essential for sonographic evaluation of the gallbladder. It promotes maximum normal distention of gallbladder. One should use a high frequency transducer. The overall gain setting must be high enough to detect the parenchymal pattern of liver and to have enough enhanced transmission of the sound distal to the gallbladder, to allow detection of acoustic shadows.

Multiple longitudinal and transverse sections through the gallbladder at 0.5 intervals in end inspiration must be performed to complete the evaluation of gallbladder.

Patient should be studied in two positions, in supine and left posterior oblique or supine and left lateral decubitus position to demonstrate movement of any gallstone with in the gallbladder. In these positions, the fundus of gallbladder is dependent which may allow a small stone obscured by the neck of the gallbladder to become visible in the fundus.

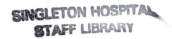

Intrahepatic bile ducts are seen as fluid filled tubular channels lying anterior to the portal vein. Generally, it is easier to identify dilated intrahepatic ducts on longitudinal scans in the right lobe of liver and of transverse scans on left lobe of liver.

Since the portal vessels enter the liver in oblique plane, oblique scans of the right upper quadrant are best for evaluating the extrahepatic biliary tree.

An oblique scanning plane combined with a left posterior oblique patient position will bring the common bile duct directly anterior to the portal vein.

It is essential that only single pass scans be used for improved resolution and for demonstration of acoustic shadowing.

Ultrasound Appearances of Gallbladder

Normal gallbladder: It is a pear-shaped with thin wall (due to stretching).

If the gallbladder is partly contracted, the wall is clearly visible. The bile is echo-free.

The tortuous cystic duct near the neck of gallbladder may cast an acoustic shadow and thus simulate a stone.

Cystic duct lies inferior to the position of portal vein. It causes moderate echogenic shadow (Figs 7.2A and B).

Gallbladder variation: Folding of gallbladder fundus (Phrygian cap) (Fig. 7.3).
Septation in gallbladder lumen (Fig. 7.4).

Gallbladder debris: In any nonfunctioning gallbladder, small mobile particles are frequently demonstrated on ultrasound image. They are thought to be minute crystals of cholesterol and bile salt may fill the gallbladder. Layering can also be seen when bile becomes inspissated or viscid, in this case the movement with change in position is slow. On ultrasound, gallbladder appears normal in size and shape.

Contents of gallbladder return low level echoes. These do not cause shadow.

Commonly they settle with gravity on change of position (Fig. 7.5).

Ascitis: The gallbladder rounds up. The wall often appear thickened (Fig. 7.6A).

Gas in gallbladder: The region of gallbladder returns high level echoes. Gas in biliary tract also produces high level echoes (Fig. 7.6B).

Gallstones: The criteria for diagnosing the presence of gallstone are:
Echogenic region within the gallbladder.

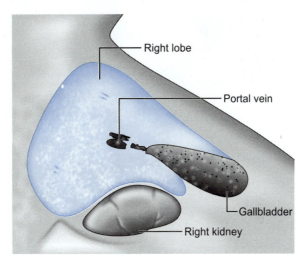

Fig. 7.2A Normal gallbladder

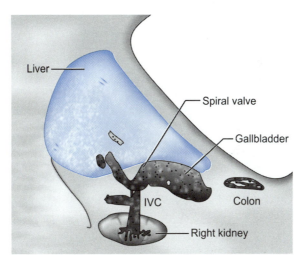

Fig. 7.2B Spiral valve

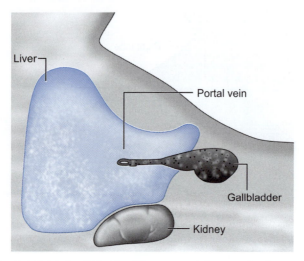

Fig. 7.3 Folded gallbladder (Phrygian cap) (Longitudinal section)

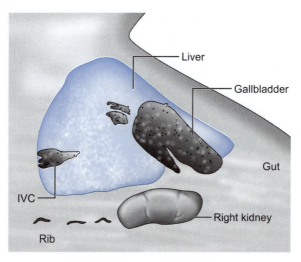

Fig. 7.4 Septate gallbladder

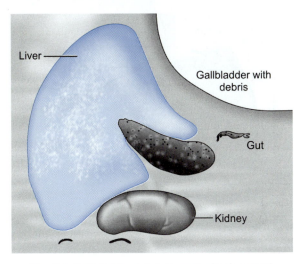

Fig. 7.5 Gallbladder debris (Longitudinal section)

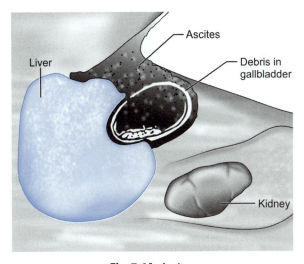

Fig. 7.6A Ascites

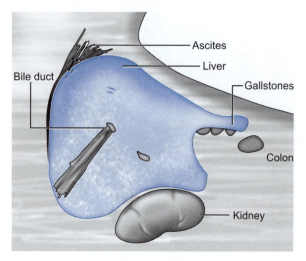

Fig. 7.6B Gas in bile duct

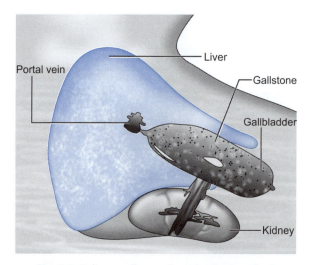

Fig. 7.7 Solitary gallstone (Longitudinal section)

Acoustic shadowing: Movement of the stone on changing the posture of the patient (postural movement) (Figs 7.7 and 7.8).

Problem arises when: Stones are impacted, usually in the neck of gallbladder (Fig. 7.9).

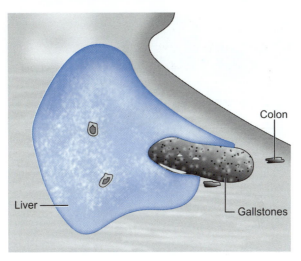

Fig. 7.8 Layered gallstones

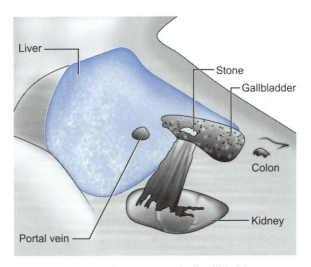

Fig. 7.9 Gallstones in neck of gallbladder

When the gallstones are occur in an empty gallbladder (Fig. 7.10). Proper fasting of patient is helpful in avoiding such a mistake. Gallbladder contracted tightly around the stones (Fig. 7.11).

Nonmobile gallstone (Figs 7.12A and B).

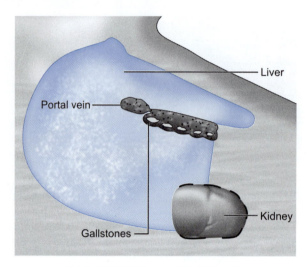

Fig. 7.10 Stone in empty gallbladder

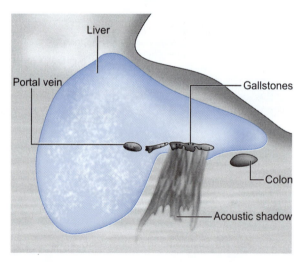

Fig. 7.11 Contracted gallbladder filled with stones (Longitudinal section)

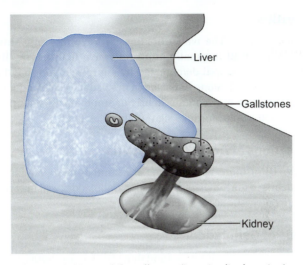

Fig. 7.12A Nonmobile gallstone (Longitudinal section)

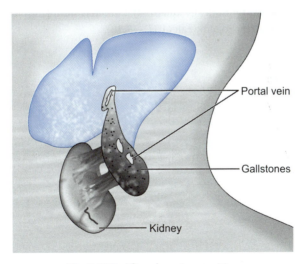

Fig. 7.12B After changing position

Cholecystitis

Acute cholecystitis: The wall thickness is beyond 4 mm thickness. The gallbladder wall is usually more reflective than nearby liver but characteristically it is well demarcated by a fine echopoor band (due to inflammatory edema). Stone impacted in cystic duct. Gallbladder contents may be echofree or may contain debris or stone. Local tenderness over gallbladder "ultrasonic Murphy's sign" (Figs 7.13A and B).

Complications of Acute Cholecystitis

Empyema: Ultrasound appearances are same as acute cholecystitis. It contains debris in the lumen of gallbladder. Gallbladder wall may rupture to form a pericholecystic abscess (Fig. 7.14).

Mucocele of Gallbladder

Gallbladder is markedly distended and thin wall. Large echofree gallbladder or may contain debris together with stone. Differential diagnosis (D/D) physiologically distended gallbladder due to prolonged fast (Fig. 7.15).

Chronic cholecystitis: Gallbladder wall is markedly thickened with strongly reflective shadows (chronically inflamed). Lumen is shrunken.

It may contain echogenic calculi (Fig. 7.16).

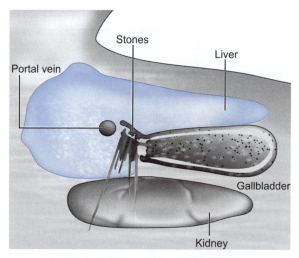

Fig. 7.13A Acute cholecystitis (Longitudinal section)

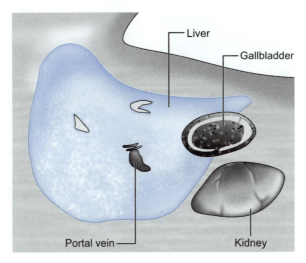

Fig. 7.13B Acute cholecystitis (Transverse section)

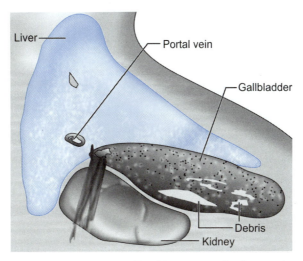

Fig. 7.14 Empyema: Gallbladder (Longitudinal section)

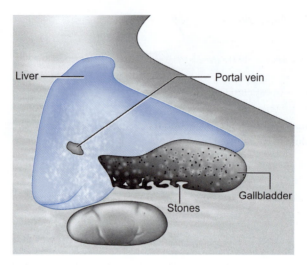

Fig. 7.15 Mucocele: Gallbladder (Longitudinal section)

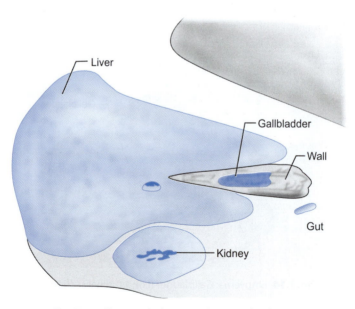

Fig. 7.16 Chronic cholecystitis (Longitudinal section)

Causes of Gallbladder Wall Thickness

- Contracted normal gallbladder
- Cholecystitis—acute, chronic
- Ascites
- Hypo albuminemia
- Adenomyomatosis
- Carcinoma—primary or secondary
- Lesion around the gallbladder.

Gallbladder polyp: Attachment of polyp in the wall of gallbladder. It is immobile. It does not cast a shadow.

D/D—Focal adenomyomatosis can produce a similar appearance (Fig. 7.17).

Carcinoma of gallbladder: Early tumor appear a polypoid mass in the lumen of gallbladder. Local invasion of liver produces a mass of low reflectivity in the region of gallbladder and porta hepatis. Commonly out line of the bladder is difficult to define. Echogenic calculi may be seen in gallbladder. Dilated bite duct (obstruction at porta hepatis) (Figs 7.18A and B).

Carcinoma of extrahepatic biliary tree: It causes irregular stricture.

The appearance of obstructive jaundice are seen.

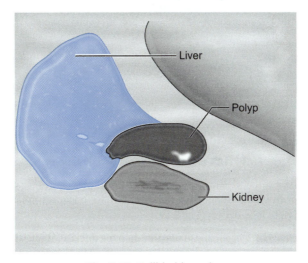

Fig. 7.17 Gallbladder polyp

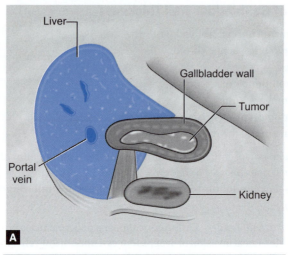

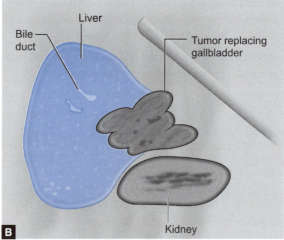

Figs 7.18A and B Carcinoma of gallbladder

Cholangiocarcinoma: Reflective ill-defined mass occupies mostly lateral portion of right lobe of liver (Fig. 7.19).

Obstruction at porta hepatis: Dilated intrahepatic ducts without extrahepatic obstruction may indicate a lesion in the porta hepatis. This is a common site for metastatic nodes (Figs 7.20 to 7.22).

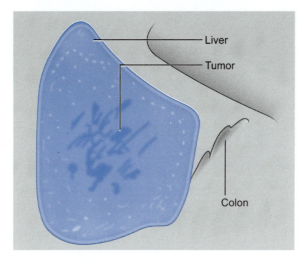

Fig. 7.19 Cholangiocarcinoma

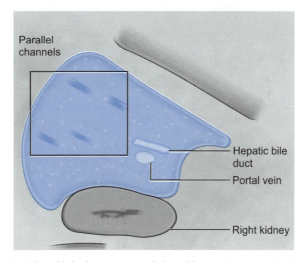

Fig. 7.20 Dilated bile ducts (minimal duct dilation) (Longitudinal section)

Obstruction at ampulla of Vater: With any biliary dilatation, the head of the pancreas should be suspected as causing a constriction.

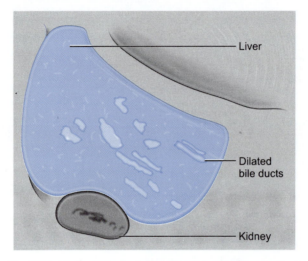

Fig. 7.21 Marked bile duct dilatation (Longitudinal section)

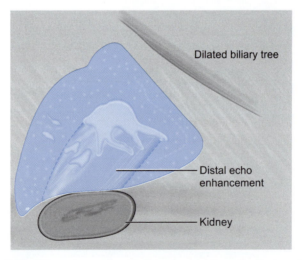

Fig. 7.22 Biliary obstruction (Stellate pattern) (Longitudinal section) (Near porta hepatis)

Jaundice

The site or cause of jaundice may be found as an intrahepatic lesion such as cirrhosis or hepatitis or an extrahepatic disease such as stones, tumor, strictures or pancreatic head pathology (Figs 7.23 to 7.25).

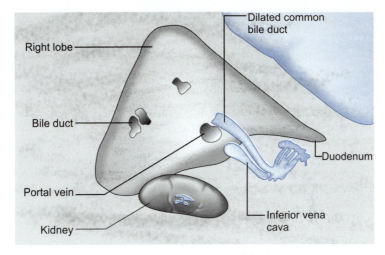

Fig. 7.23 Stone in common bile duct

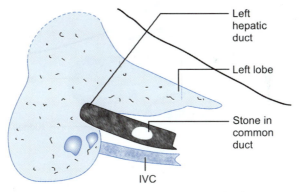

Fig. 7.24 Stone in common duct (Longitudinal section)

Choledochal Cysts

It is localized cystic dilatation of common bile duct. It occurs during first two decades of life. Intermittent symptoms are occurring when cyst distends and compress common bile duct causes jaundice, pain and a mass.

Ultrasound findings are normal gallbladder, dilated cystic duct, normal or dilated common bile duct.

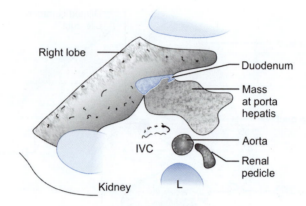

Fig. 7.25 Obstructed common bile duct (Transverse section)

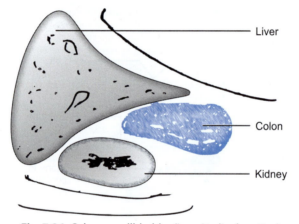

Fig. 7.26 Colon as gallbladder (Longitudinal section)

Colon

Sometimes colonic shadow between liver and right kidney can give a false impression of gallbladder, containing calculi. Careful scanning will show peristalsis (Fig. 7.26).

8

Pancreas

Anatomy

This roughly fish-shaped organ lies behind the stomach, with its head and neck in the C-shaped curve of the duodenum, body extending horizontally across the posterior abdominal wall, and its tail touching the spleen. It is curved around the superior mesenteric vessels. The head fits into the concavity of the duodenum, the neck lies in front of the beginning of the portal vein below the pyloric opening of the stomach and above the superior mesenteric vessels. The body drapes over the midline superior to the aorta, traveling in front of left kidney and adrenal area and under the stomach. The body tapers to form the tail which usually touches the spleen just below the hilum. This gland varies in size according to sex and individuals, being larger in the male than in the female. Roughly 12–18 cm in length, 2–3 cm wide and approximately 1 cm thick, the pancreas weighs about 3 ounce (oz) (Fig. 8.1).

Structure

The pancreas is one of the most important organs of the body. Pancreatic structure resembles that of the salivary glands; although the pancreas has no capsule, portions of connective tissue divide it into lobes and lobules composed of cells which pour these secretions into microscopic ducts. These tiny ducts unite to form larger ducts which eventually join the main pancreatic duct 'duct of Wirsung' which extends the entire length of the gland. It empties into the duodenum at the same point as the common bile duct 'ampulla of Vater'. In addition to cells which secrete into the pancreatic ducts, numerous clusters of cells are found scattered throughout the pancreas. These cell clusters are called islets or islands of Langerhans. They also are glands but their secretion 'insulin' passes into the bloodstream rather than ducts. In other words, the islands of Langerhans are microscopic-ductless, endocrine glands. Diabetes mellitus results from the degeneration of these cells.

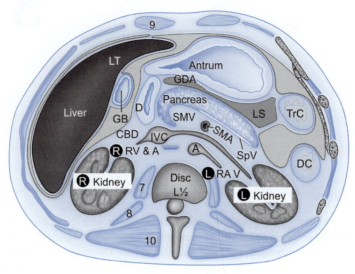

Fig. 8.1 Pancreas and its relation with visceras and retroperitoneal vessels
Abbreviations: A, aorta; CBD, common bile duct; D, duodenum; DC, descending colon; GB, gallbladder; GDA, gastroduodenal artery; LRA and V, left renal artery and vein; LS, lesser sac; LT, ligamentum teres; SMA, superior mesenteric artery; SMV, superior mesenteric vein; SpV, splenic vein; TrC, transverse colon

Diseases of the Pancreas (Fig. 8.2)

In sclerosis, atrophy, acute and chronic inflammatory changes and new growths in the pancreas, and absence or lessening of pancreatic secretion may be evident. Hemorrhage into the pancreas can cause death and *acute hemorrhagic pancreatitis* is a combination of inflammation and hemorrhage in which the pancreas is enlarged and infiltrated with blood. Violent pain, vomiting and collapse are the chief features. This latter condition is usually treated with surgery and is followed by recovery. Hemorrhagic inflammation may be followed by gangrene of the pancreas which is usually fatal. *Chronic pancreatitis* occurs in connection with symptoms of catarrhal jaundice which may due to the pressure of the swollen pancreas on the common bile duct. The organ is enlarged, very hard and the symptoms are pain, dyspepsia, jaundice, weight loss and the presence of fat in the stools. This latter sign is common to all pancreatic disease. The pancreas, like other organs is subject to the occurrence of new growths, tumors and cysts, syphilis and TB. Of these, carcinoma of the head or the organ is the most common. Fibrosis and calcification of the organ are common byproduct of chronic pancreatitis. *Acute pancreatitis*

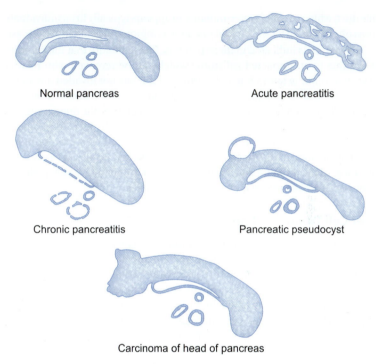

Normal pancreas

Acute pancreatitis

Chronic pancreatitis

Pancreatic pseudocyst

Carcinoma of head of pancreas

Fig. 8.2 Pancreatic pathology as seen by ultrasound imaging

may be due to the regurgitation of bile into the pancreatic ducts, or it may be hematogenous in origin. The most severe types of this infection may produce marked local hemorrhage and the enzymes liberated may cause marked necrosis of the fat in the adjacent parts of the abdominal cavity. The disease usually comes on suddenly with severe abdominal pain (often radiating through to the back) and vomiting. The temperature may be elevated and usually the condition is mistakenly diagnosed as 'acute indigestion'.

Tumors in Head of Pancreas

Tumors in this region are detected by the fact that they obstruct the common bile duct where it passes through the head of the pancreas to join the pancreatic duct, and empty at the ampulla of Vater into the duodenum. Obstruction to the flow of bile produces jaundice, clay-colored stools and dark urine. This disease usually occurs in older, thin man. It must be differentiated from jaundice due to a biliary obstruction caused by a gallstone in the common bile duct, which usually is intermittent and appears typically in fat individuals, most often women who have had previous symptoms of gallbladder disease.

Operation is indicated in these patients, first to be sure that the jaundice is not due to an impacted gallstone, which can be removed with relative ease. If a tumor is found it may be removed if it has not invaded any of the important structures adjacent to it (portal vein, superior mesenteric artery). The operation entails removal of the head of the pancreas, the duodenum and adjacent stomach and the distal part of the common bile duct. The stomach, the cut end of the pancreas and the common bile duct then are anastomoses and may be done in one or two stages. It has resulted in cure in many cases of cancer of the ampulla and the bile ducts, but is apparently only palliative in most cases of cancer of the head of the pancreas.

Islet Cell Tumors of Pancreas

Located in the pancreas are the islets of Langerhans, small nests of cells which secrete directly into the bloodstream and are therefore part of the glands of internal secretion (endocrines). The secretion, insulin is involved in sugar metabolism and a deficient secretion produces diabetes. Tumors of these cells produce a hypersecretion of insulin so that body sugar is used up too rapidly resulting in the fall of blood sugar hypoglycemia. Islet tumors are corrected by surgery. They may be benign adenomas or they may be malignant. Complete removal usually results in a dramatic cure. Occasionally the symptoms are produced by simple hypertrophy of this tissue rather than tumor. In this case a partial pancreatectomy is indicated (removal of tail and part of the body).

Physiology of the Pancreas

The pancreas is found in the midabdomen behind the stomach in front of the spine in an overcrowded space of assorted organs including the liver, kidneys and large intestine. A very busy organ, the pancreas helps supply the fuel to stoke cellular fires.

In actuality the pancreas is two glands wrapped in one package. It produces two hormones that empty into the bloodstream. *Glucose*, or blood sugar provides the fuel for cells; *insulin* controls the delicate and critical task of keeping the blood sugar at proper levels and sees that it is properly burned.

Without the enzymes the pancreas produces the body could consume enormous quantities of food and still be malnourished.

The key role of the pancreas in digestion is to produce two pints of digestive juices each day. Imagine 32 oz. of fluids from a 3 oz gland; when food leaves the stomach it is in a highly acid state, the consistency of gruel, and called *chyme*. This acid acts in breaking down proteins. It could spell disaster further along the digestive tract by eating away the delicate lining of the small intestine except for the alkaline pancreatic juices that neutralize this acid.

The pancreas also plays a key role in rendering ingested food, acceptable to the body.

To accomplish this feat the pancreas produces 3 enzymes.

1. *Trysin:* To break down proteins to amino acids for use in building body tissues.
2. *Amylase:* To convert starch into sugar.
3. *Lipase:* To attack fat globules, breaking them down into fatty acids and glycerin.

In the event that the total production of digestive juices by the pancreas was destroyed, saliva and gastric and intestinal secretions would do a minimal job but digestion would be a misery.

Insulin production is the most critical task of the pancreas.

Under-production of insulin results in diabetes. To produce insulin approximately a million 'Islet' cells are scattered through the pancreas, each an independent little factory.

The trillions of cells that comprise the body are very efficient miniature furnaces burning glucose to generate energy. Insulin sees to it that they receive the precise amount of fuel required.

Insulin also plays a role in helping cells burn glucose. If the islets shut down the cells would try to burn other fuels. Fat would be burned and protein would be drained from muscles to provide energy. The body would become cadaverously thin, insatiably hungry and constantly thirsty. Unable to burn the sugar, it would be excreted to 'sweetish' urine, in quantities as high as 4 gls/day. These are the symptoms of diabetes.

Insulin also affects the liver. It is the liver that is the storehouse of any excess glucose that may be circulating in the blood. As blood passes through the liver it is stimulated by insulin to convert the excess into a starchy substance called *glycogen,* which is then stored till needed. When the need arises the glycogen is converted back into glucose and fed into the blood.

By consuming sweets in excessive amounts this delicate balance goes out of kilter, causing a step-up in insulin production, increasing the fires of cellular combustion. This is the reason a candy bar is a good source of energy. Conversely, when blood sugar drops too low, insulin production is cut in effect banking the fire.

Additionally, the pancreas presents other problems. It is the 'phantom' organ because its location makes visualization so difficult and the symptoms of pancreatic disease mimic so many other conditions. Surgeons have a difficult time getting at the pancreas without injuring neighboring organs.

Another common problem is *acute pancreatitis*. The cause of this inflammation are many viz., trauma, alcoholic abuse, arterial disease, etc. One of the most common causes is a result of poor 'plumbing'. The pancreas shares with the liver and gallbladder the common exit duct into the duodenum and bile from the liver can backup into the pancreatic duct system, injuring or destroying it. A gallstone may also block the exit duct, backing up enzymes which then begin digesting the pancreas itself. If this condition persists over a long period of time it is usually fatal. Indeed over 2500 persons die annually as a result of acute pancreatitis. One can live without the pancreas because artificial hormones are available to replace those that would be missing, but the quality of life is not very comfortable.

The pancreas is prey to a variety of tumors. One of the worst is the *adenoma* that causes over-production of insulin. Cancer of the pancreas carries a grave prognosis and ranks 3rd after lung and colon-rectum cancer, as a killer gallbladder disease and cystic fibrosis may also result in pancreatic involvement.

Fact and Fallacies in Evaluation of Pancreas

Gray scale ultrasound is known to be a reliable method for identifying the normal pancreas through the use of known vascular structures surrounding the gland. The splenic vein and superior mesenteric vein are still the major landmarks used to identify the pancreas. The pancreas itself varies not only in shape but also in orientation in the abdomen from almost transverse to a nearly vertical orientation. Careful understanding and observation of the surrounding anatomy will reduce the risk of error when the orientation of the gland varies greatly from the typical (Figs 8.3 to 8.7).

Discussion

In the transverse plane the splenic vein is probably the easiest landmark to identify and is the point at which to begin detailed examination of the pancreas. The splenic vein is found in most cases along the posterosuperior aspect of the pancreas, identifying the body and tail of that organ. At or just below this level the confluence of the superior mesenteric and splenic veins may also be seen. The portal vein is seen cephalad to this level. Head of the pancreas frequently lies inferior to the main branch of the portal vein, the neck of the pancreas being usually more in proximity to the portal vein. The inferior location of the pancreatic head has been well documented and can best be observed in sagittal section anterior to the inferior vena cava. We have observed great variability in the distance between the portal vein and

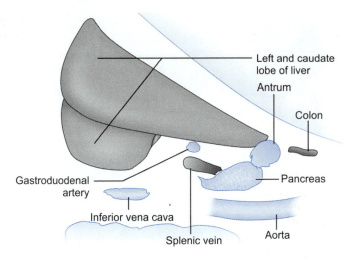

Fig. 8.3 Normal pancreas (Longitudinal section)

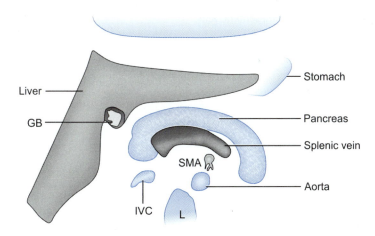

Fig. 8.4 Normal pancreas (Transverse section)
Abbreviations: GB, gallbladder; IVC, inferior vena cava;
SMA, superior mesenteric artery

the head of the pancreas since the portal vein curves superiorly toward the
liver hilus and the pancreatic head may curve quite inferiorly.

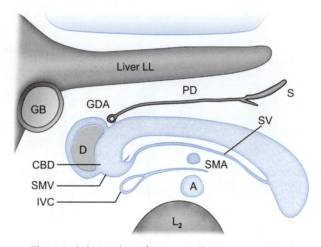

Fig. 8.5 Relationship of pancreas (Transverse section)
(Where splenic vein joins superior mesenteric vein)
Abbreviations: A, aorta; CBD, common bile duct; D, duodenum; GB, gallbladder;
GDA, gastroduodenal artery; IVC, inferior vena cava; SMA, superior mesenteric
artery; SMV, superior mesenteric vein

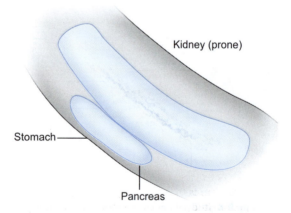

Fig. 8.6 Tail of pancreas (Longitudinal section)

When examining very thin or elderly patients when liver extends far
below the costal margin and the pancreas also appears caudad, as low as
the umbilicus.

The bile duct appear anterior to portal vein, as it leaves the liver and slopes
posteriorly towards the pancreatic head. This should not be confused with

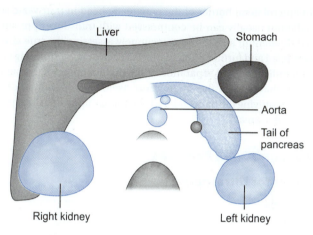

Fig. 8.7 Tail of pancreas (Transverse section)

gastroduodenal artery which also lies on the right lateral border of head of pancreas but is anterior to common bile duct and travel horizontally towards the pancreatic head.

The common bile duct lies along the posterolateral border of pancreatic head at or near the pancreatic duodenal interface, while gastroduodenal artery is found more anteriorly defining the anterolateral margin of gland.

The superior mesenteric vein has been used as landmark for the junction of head and body of pancreas. The superior mesenteric vein does not course through the pancreas but is embedded within it between the head and the uncinate process towards its junctions with the splenic vein.

The left renal vein also may be observed at the level of the body of the pancreas extending from the inferior vena cava, crossing the midline between the aorta and superior mesenteric artery toward the left kidney. This is the only normal vessel that crosses between the aorta and the superior mesenteric artery. The left renal vein is best seen in transverse section. It can also be frequently seen on longitudinal view. The superior mesenteric artery will be demonstrated in all transverse sections of the pancreas, it should be noted that the origin of the superior mesenteric artery can be somewhat superior to the pancreas and travels inferior to it, not necessarily pinpointing the location of the pancreas.

Not only are vascular structures around the pancreas useful in accurately locating the gland but the duodenum can be demonstrated and used for localization purposes. The duodenum can be observed curving around

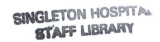

the right anterolateral border of the pancreatic head in transverse section. The duodenum usually can be compressed with transducer pressure. The collapsed duodenum aids in more accurately assessing the true size of the pancreatic head and further reduces the risk of error in interpreting bowel as a mass. Identification and separation of the duodenum from the pancreatic head has probably been the single most useful 'new' landmark in more accurately identifying the pancreas and in eliminating error in interpretation of masses in this area.

Ultrasonography of Pancreas

Indications for Ultrasound

- Pancreatitis
- Pseudocyst
- Suspected carcinoma
- Unexplained abdominal pain and weight loss.

Anatomy

Quite variable in shape and location.

Head: Medial to liver, lies in descending portion of duodenum

Body: Posterior to stomach

Tail: Goes toward hilum of spleen or just superior to upper pole of left kidney

IVC, aorta, SMA: Posterior to pancreas

Splenic vein: Along superior border of pancreas.

Ductal System

Duct of Wirsung (Main pancreatic duct)
Duct of Santorini (Accessory pancreatic duct).

Physiology

Both an endocrine and exocrine gland
Acinar cells = Exocrine functions
Islet cells = Endocrine functions
Major enzymes of digestion
- Amylase

- Trypsin
- Lipase.

Other Means of Evaluating Pancreas

Plain Abdomen Films

Calcifications—may indicate previous inflammations.
Mass—may see outline of mass as well as what it displaces, e.g. ascites.

Upper GI Series

Inflammatory changes in descending portion of duodenum if there is lesion in head of pancreas. Displacement of stomach and duodenum by pancreatic mass.

Hypotonic duodenography: Air contrast exam of duodenum of mucosal detail.

Isotope scans: Not reliable.

Arteriography: Invasive procedure; often technically difficult.

ERCP: Endoscopic retrograde cholangiopancreatography 15% failure rate.

Pancreatitis: It can be acute or chronic.

Etiology: Alcoholism, trauma, biliary tract disease.

Symptoms: Epigastric pain, nausea and vomiting, abdominal tenderness and distention.

Lab: Elevated amylase, elevated white blood cell count.

X-ray findings: Related to mass displacing other organs.

Carcinoma of pancreas: Usually occurs in 50–60 years of age 2 times more common in diabetics.

Symptoms and signs: Dull epigastric pain increased by eating, jaundice, rapid weight loss, nausea and vomiting, enlarged liver and gallbladder.

Head of pancreas most common site: It will see deformed duodenum on upper gastrointestinal (UGI). May invade common bile duct and obstruct it with resultant jaundice.

Carcinoma in body or tail: Constant pain, migratory thrombophlebitis.

Prognosis poor: Usually only palliative procedures are possible.

Pancreas: Technique

Overnight fasting is necessary for adequate evaluation. The highest frequency transducer usually 3.5 MHz, should be adjusted to display low amplitude echoes in the liver but no echoes in prevertebral vasculature when using the fluid filled stomach technique. A shallower TGC curve and decreased overall gain are usually required.

Initial scanning is performed in longitudinal and transverse plane. In end inspiration the left lobe of liver may provide a gas free acoustic shadow.

After standard longitudinal and transverse scans, oblique scans along the long axis of pancreas may be obtained.

The region of tail of pancreas is visualized by prone longitudinal scans through the upper pole of left kidney. Frequently even with adequate patient preparation, the region of pancreas is obscured by bowel gas. Twelve to eighteen oz of fluid can be administered to the patient and pancreas may be visualized through the fluid filled stomach. The patient is initially studied in left posterior oblique (LPO) position to visualize the body and tail of pancreas through the anterior abdominal wall. This position allows air with in the stomach to rise toward the antrum of the stomach. The head of the pancreas is best studied in the right posterior oblique (RPO) position with the gas rising to the fundus of stomach.

ULTRASOUND APPEARANCES

Pancreas

Normal Pancreas

Normal pancreas returns higher level of echoes than liver. This is in cases of adults.

In children the pancreas is usually less echogenic and also relatively larger.

In elderly person it is a small echogenic pancreas. This is secondary to fibrosis and atrophy that are normally found with increasing years.

Acute Pancreatitis

Diffuse enlargement of pancreas is seen. Low level of echo are visible. Margin of pancreas are blurred (Figs 8.8 and 8.9).

Hemorrhagic Pancreatitis

Pancreas is grossly enlarged. There can be prominent irregular regions within it which return a very low level of echoes and show marked distal

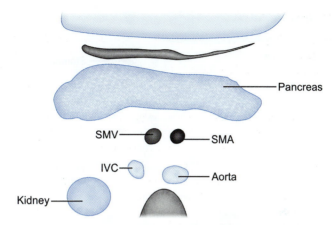

Fig. 8.8 Acute pancreatitis (Transverse section) (diffuse enlargement)
Abbreviations: IVC, Inferior vena cava; SMA, superior mesenteric artery;
SMV, superior mesenteric vein

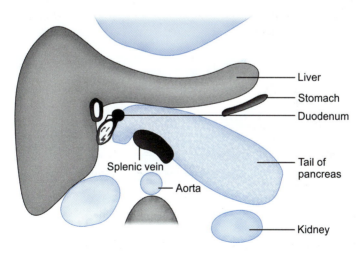

Fig. 8.9 Acute pancreatitis tail (Transverse section)

echo enhancement. The fluid features are due to hemorrhagic necrosis, debris, accounting for low level echoes within the fluid region (Figs 8.10 and 8.11).

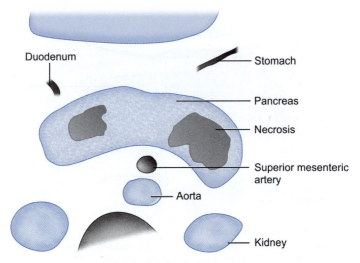

Fig. 8.10 Hemorrhagic pancreatitis (Transverse section)

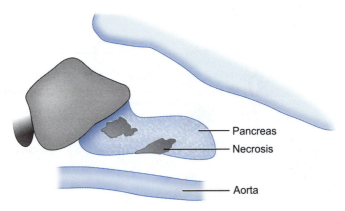

Fig. 8.11 Hemorrhagic pancreatitis (Longitudinal section)

Chronic Pancreatitis

The small pancreas returns a high level of echoes compared with adjacent liver. The high level echoes are due to fibrosis or calcification. Focal low echoes (due to ongoing inflammation) can be seen (Figs 8.12 and 8.13).

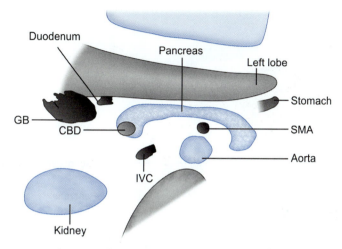

Fig. 8.12 Chronic pancreatitis (Transverse section)
Abbreviations: CBD, common bile duct; GB, gallbladder; IVC, inferior vena cava; SMA, superior mesenteric artery

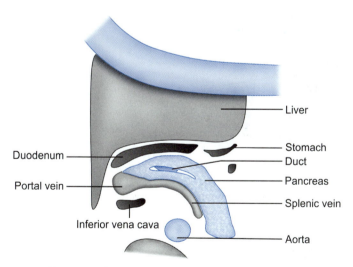

Fig. 8.13 Chronic pancreatitis (Longitudinal section)

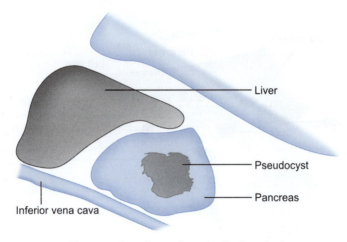

Fig. 8.14 Pseudocyst (Longitudinal section)

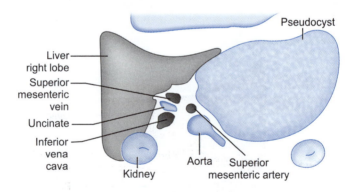

Fig. 8.15 Pseudocyst (Transverse section)

Pseudocyst

Fluid filled space (anechoic), most common near the pancreas, but may be anywhere in the abdomen. Margins are ill defined, progressing to clear cut

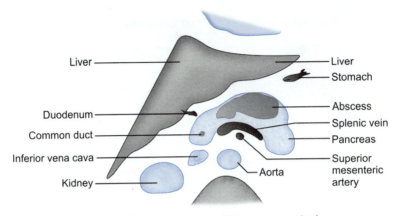

Fig. 8.16 Pancreatic abscess (Transverse section)

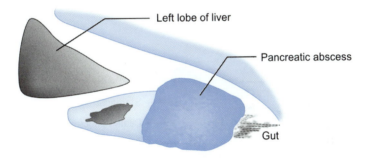

Fig. 8.17 Pancreatic abscess (Longitudinal section)

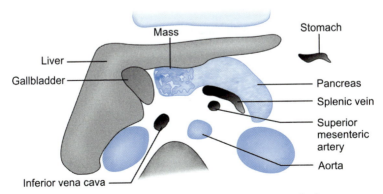

Fig. 8.18 Pancreatic carcinoma (Transverse section)

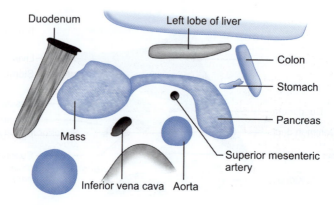

Fig. 8.19 Carcinoma of head of pancreas (Transverse section)

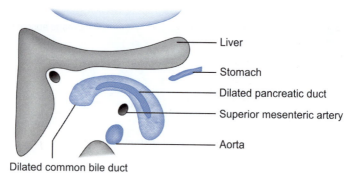

Fig. 8.20 Carcinoma of ampulla

margins as it matures. The pancreatic tissue surrounding the cyst shows low reflectivity. Spontaneous regression of pseudocyst can be seen in some cases (Figs 8.14 and 8.15).

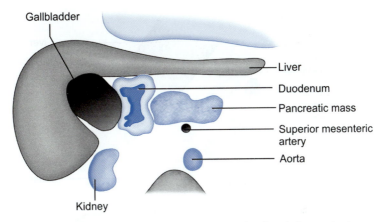

Fig. 8.21 Carcinoma of head of pancreas (duodenal obstruction)

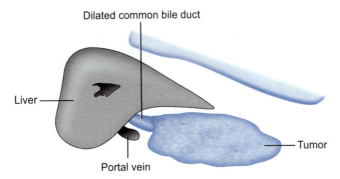

Fig. 8.22 Carcinoma of head and body of pancreas (Longitudinal section)

Pancreatic Abscess

Large mass in the region of pancreas returns a predominantly low level of echoes with some degree of distal enhancement. There are however, regions of medium and high level echoes (Figs 8.16 and 8.17).

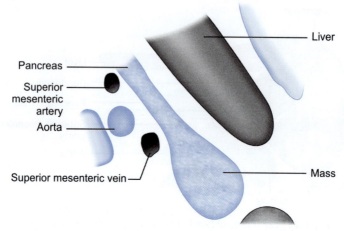

Fig. 8.23 Carcinoma of tail of pancreas (Transverse section)

Pancreatic Carcinoma

Irregular focal mass, predominantly low level echoes. Obstruction of common bile duct and pancreatic duct can lead to the dilatation of common bile duct and pancreatic duct.

Nodal and liver metastases can be seen (Figs 8.18 to 8.23).

9

Abdominal Aorta

Introduction

It begins its route at 12 thoracic vertebra and carries oxygenated blood to the tissue of body for their nutrition. In the average individual it ends at L4 vertebra. At this point aorta divides into the right and left common iliac arteries. The area of bifurcation may be indicated on the surface of abdomen by a point about 2.5 cm below and slightly to the left of umbilicus (Figs 9.1 and 9.2).

In an adult the normal diameter of lumen is approximately 25 mm at xiphoid level. The lumen decreases uniformly to approximately 15 mm at the bifurcation of aorta.

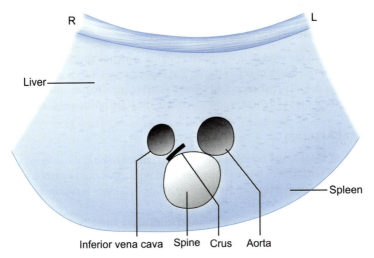

Fig. 9.1 Normal aorta (Transverse section)

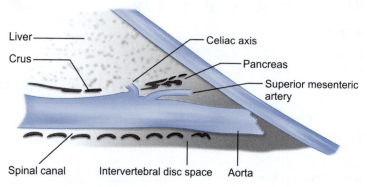

Fig. 9.2 Normal aorta (Longitudinal section)

Celiac Axis

The first main branch of abdominal aorta, and largest branch in diameter. It arises as short thick trunk 8–40 mm in length from anterior aspect of aorta. It gives three branches.

1. Left gastric artery
2. Common hepatic artery
3. Splenic artery.

Superior Mesenteric Artery

It arises from the level of first lumbar vertebra which is approximately 5–15 mm below the origin of celiac trunk. The superior mesenteric artery (SMA) originates dorsal to pancreas and splenic vein emerges to run anterior to the uncinate process of pancreas and anterior to the third portion of duodenum.

Renal Arteries

The right renal artery is longer than left and passes behind the inferior vena cava. Left renal artery is usually higher than right. Anterior to each artery is corresponding renal vein, and posteriorly at hilus of kidney is commencement of ureter.

Middle suprarenal arteries come off from aorta laterally and pass a little above the renal arteries to suprarenal organs.

Vascular Pathology

Atherosclerosis

In aorta, atherosclerosis usually occurs distal to renal arteries and actual occlusion is usually secondary to thrombosis. When occlusion takes place in any artery blood supply to organ is generally taken over by the collateral circulation.

Aneurysm

Abnormal dilatation of a vessel wall due to weakness in the wall or a congenital defect. There are three main types of aneurysm (Figs 9.3 and 9.4).

Dissecting aneurysm occurs when blood make its way between the layers of a vessel wall. This type of aneurysm always arises in thoracic aorta. Fusiforms are usually atherosclerotic in nature and most often occurs distal to renal arteries. Saccular aneurysm will not involve the entire circumference but will yield to a weak patch on one side of vessel. This type is usually caused by trauma.

Splenic artery aneurysm are fairly common. They may or may not be calcified.

Aneurysms of both celiac and superior mesenteric arteries are most likely syphilitic or mycotic in nature.

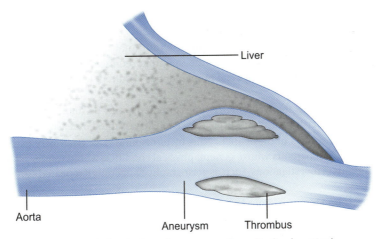

Fig. 9.3 Abdominal aortic aneurysm (Longitudinal section)

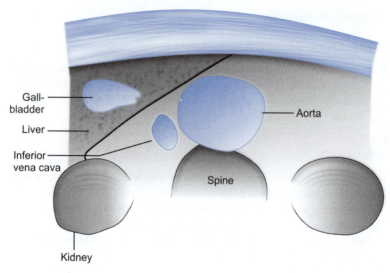

Fig. 9.4 Abdominal aortic aneurysm (Transverse section)

Ultrasound

Limitation in resolution of ultrasound examinations are bowel gas, barium, nonfocused transducer. Proper transducer selection is very important for optimal detail. Generally the greatest resolution is possible in thin to medium patients with a 3.5 MHz transducer with surface diameter of 13 mm. Simple sector scans are preferable to linear scan.

The diagnosis and assessment of abdominal aortic aneurysms by ultrasound examination has become the preferred method of choice. It is noninvasive study so no special preparation is required. It shows the entire aneurysm.

One can see the wall of aorta, measurements may be made that aid in prediction of rupture and if surgical excision is warranted or feasible.

Serial studies of these aneurysms by ultrasound have been very useful especially in patients whose general physical condition would render other methods of investigations, such as aortography dangerous if repeated several times.

Ultrasound however, does have restrictions:

- Inadequate view of some of smaller branches of aorta.
- The SMA and renal arteries can usually be seen but not always well enough to determine their normality. Stenosis or narrowing of these arteries

usually cannot be seen, nor can small atherosclerotic plaque on the aortic wall.

Both transverse and longitudinal scans are performed with patient in supine position.

When aorta is markedly tortuous as it often is in older patients, it is best to start with transverse scans. The course of aorta can be marked at mid point of patient skin with a wax pencil. At the completion of transverse scans the marks are connected and longitudinal oblique scans are performed. It is not always possible to record the full length of vessel on one scan.

Localized fluid collections adjacent to aortic aneurysm may be suggestive of retroperitoneal hemorrhage. Free intra-abdominal fluid in association with aneurysm may also lead to a diagnosis of rupture.

The aorta, SMA, celiac artery, renal arteries, proximal portion of hepatic and splenic arteries are visualized in transverse scan: starting at xiphoid and going caudal at 5 mm to 1 cm intervals, all these structures are important boundary landmarks for cephalic and posterior aspect of pancreas. On longitudinal scans the celiac and SMA can usually be seen arising from aorta. The body of pancreas is anterior to SMA. This artery being routinely used landmark (Fig. 9.2).

The hepatic artery and splenic artery if visualized, are excellent cephalic boundaries of the body of pancreas.

One may use the SMA as a landmark in locating the renal arteries in transverse scans, since they usually originate at approximately the same level.

Spleen

Physiology

The spleen is a purple, concave, delicate structure tucked under the diaphragm on the left side adjacent to the 10th rib. It is an organ of the lymphatic system consisting of organized masses of encapsulated lymphatic tissue intimately associated with blood sinusoids and other vessels. In effect, the spleen filters blood. The spleen manufactured lymphocytes and monocytes for export and is very active in immune response to the presence of antigens (microorganisms, etc.). Its macrophages remove debris from the blood and specifically break down aged red blood corpuscles. The heme portion of the hemoglobin molecule is converted indirectly into bilirubin, which is conducted to the liver by way of hepatic portal vein and incorporated into the manufacture of bile. In fact, it is largely responsible for the yellow color of bile. Accumulation of bilirubin in the blood is jaundice and is generally indicative of liver or gallbladder disease. The storage function of red corpuscles in the spleen is generally considered to be minimal.

Spleen: Technique

Air in stomach obscures visualization of spleen in supine position. A 3.5 MHz transducer with a medium or long focal length is most often used. The gain setting should be adjusted to demonstrate the parenchymal echoes of spleen with an intensity similar to that used for liver. It is best to obtain scan in deep inspiration.

The best images are usually obtained with the patient in right lateral decubitus position, in longitudinal scan in coronal plane.

Transverse scans are obtained from the level of diaphragm caudally.

Usually longitudinal and transverse scans at 1 cm intervals are sufficient for evaluation of spleen.

Ultrasound Appearances

Spleen

On ultrasound the spleen returns mid gray echoes of an even texture that are similar to liver in texture but are lower in intensity. Scanty vascular structures can be made toward the hilum where the larger venous and occasional arterial branch can be seen (Figs 10.1 and 10.2).

Spleen with Pleural Effusion

The crescentic pattern of effusion on transverse section is characteristic. In this projection the diaphragm is prominent. Strong echoes are obtained from fluid lung interface (Figs 10.3 and 10.4).

Subphrenic Abscess

Anechoic lesion with low level echoes are visible. The collection usually fluid with thickened capsule which is suggestive of an abscess (differential diagnosis hematoma). It is very difficult to differentiate the subphrenic abscess from splenic abscess (Figs 10.5 and 10.6).

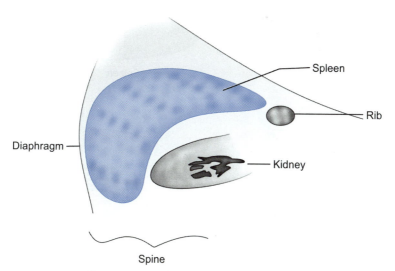

Fig. 10.1 Normal spleen (Transverse section)

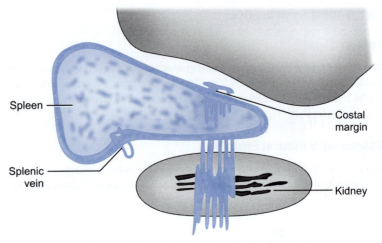

Fig. 10.2 Normal spleen (Longitudinal section)

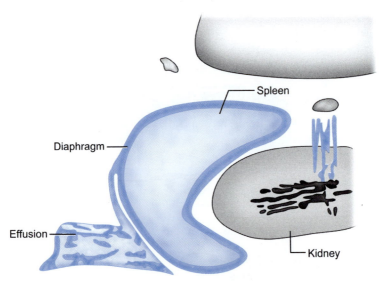

Fig. 10.3 Left pleural effusion (Transverse section)

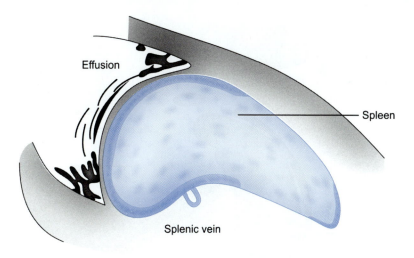

Fig. 10.4 Pleural effusion (Longitudinal section)

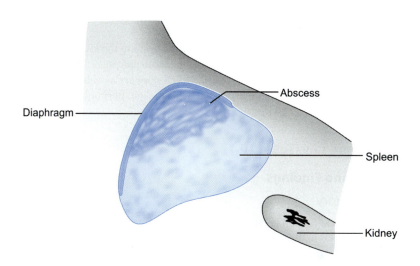

Fig. 10.5 Left subphrenic abscess (Transverse section)

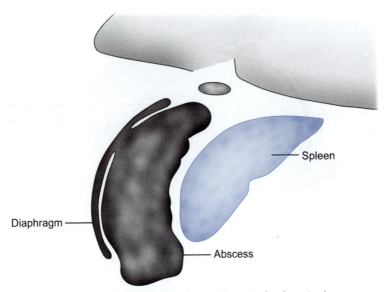

Fig. 10.6 Subphrenic abscess (Longitudinal section)

Masses Near Spleen

Normal nearby structures that can cause confusion are the kidney, portion of gut mainly stomach, local spread from malignant spleen.

Splenic trauma leads to hematoma which appears as echo poor zone either with in the spleen or adjacent to it. Leakage into peritonium gives the typical appearance of ascites.

Splenomegaly (Table 10.1)

Ultrasound Findings

Inflammatory

Acute malaria: Spleen is moderately enlarged with a uniform echotexture. The echo levels in the spleen are low, compared with those of liver.

Active tuberculosis: There is moderate splenomegaly with in near uniform echotexture. The echo level is slightly lower than liver. Associated pleural effusion may be there (Fig. 10.7).

Old tuberculosis: The spleen may show small highly reflective foci which are either fibrotic or calcific. Spleen may be moderately or grossly enlarged with varying echolevels most often of medium or high intensity (Fig. 10.8).

Table 10.1 Etiology of splenomegaly

Inflammatory	Malaria Tuberculosis
Infiltratory	Amyloid
Congestive	Congestive heart failure Portal hypertension
Hematological	Polycythemia vera
Neoplastic	Leukemia Lymphomas
Focal disorders	Cyst Abscess Malignant lymphoreticular metastatic

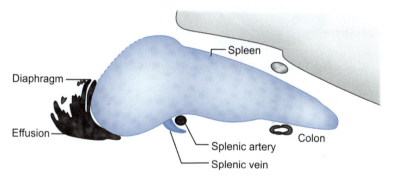

Fig. 10.7 Tuberculosis (Transverse section) active

Hematological

Polycythemia and Sickle Cell Anemia

The spleen is moderately to grossly enlarged with a medium echo intensity (Fig. 10.9).

Repeated infarcts in sickle cell anemia leads to atrophy of spleen and medium echo intensity is replaced by strong refractive scar.

Congestive

- Congestive heart failure
- Portal hypertension

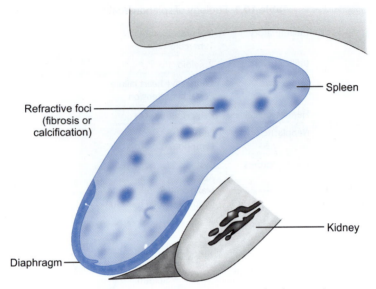

Fig. 10.8 Tuberculosis chronic (Longitudinal section)

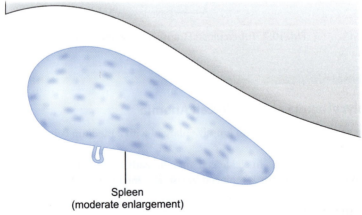

Fig. 10.9 Polycythemia (Transverse section)

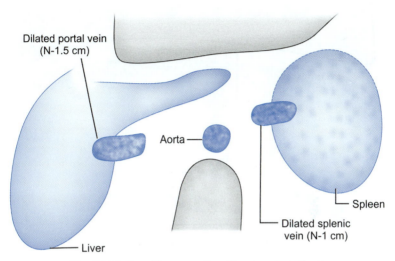

Fig. 10.10 Portal hypertension (Transverse section)

Spleen is moderately enlarged. It shows medium level of echoes. Dilatation of splenic vein can be demonstrated at the hilum (Fig. 10.10).

Malignant

Acute leukemia: The spleen shows moderate splenomegaly with low level echoes, as in acute sepsis (Fig. 10.11).

Chronic leukemia: Large spleen with uniform echotexture. The spleen shows low level echoes.

Lymphomas: Moderate to severe degree of splenomegaly is seen. The echopattern may be low level echoes as compared to liver or relatively anechoic spleen. There may be upper abdomen lymphadenopathy (Para-aortic, mesenteric, splenic) (Figs 10.12 and 10.13).

Focal Disorders

Cyst: It is anechoic. The cyst may be small or large. On ultrasound (in large cyst) the precise diagnosis of tissue of origin cannot be made from retroperitoneal cyst, pseudocyst of pancreas and large cyst of upper pole of kidney (Fig. 10.14).

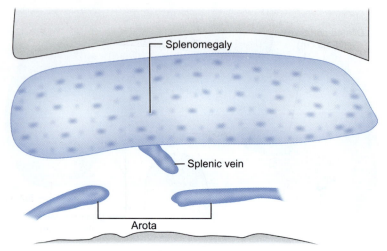

Fig. 10.11 Leukemia (Longitudinal section)

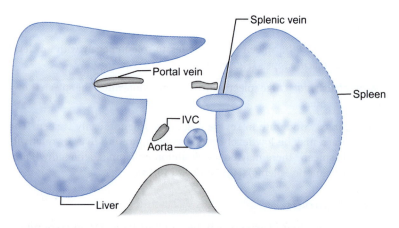

Fig. 10.12 Lymphoma—chronic myeloid leukemia (Transverse section)

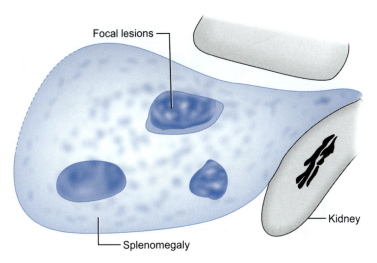

Fig. 10.13 Focal lymphoma (Longitudinal section)

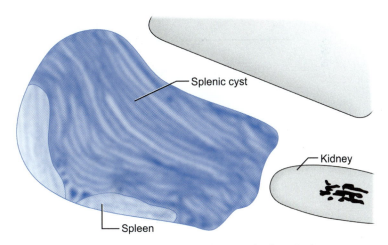

Fig. 10.14 Splenic cyst (Longitudinal section)

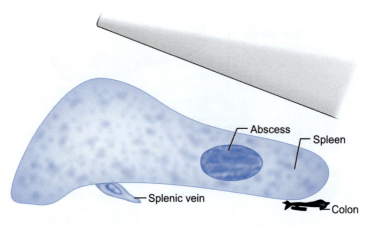

Fig. 10.15 Splenic abscess (Longitudinal section)

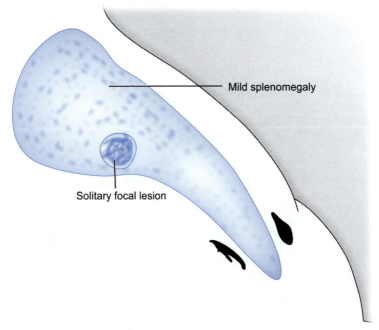

Fig. 10.16 Hodgkin's disease (Longitudinal section)

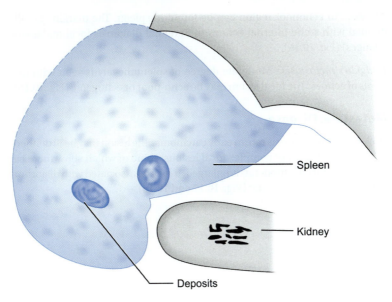

Fig. 10.17 Splenic metastases (Transverse section)

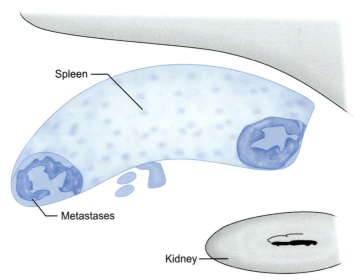

Fig. 10.18 Splenic metastases (Longitudinal section)

Abscess: An echopoor region can be found in spleen. The margins are ill-defined with some internal echoes (differential diagnosis focal malignant changes) (Fig. 10.15).

Hodgkin's metastases: Moderate degree of splenomegaly is seen with low levels of echoes. The focal lesion may be echo-poor or echogenic (Fig. 10.16).

Metastatic Disease

The splenic metastases is rare in early carcinoma. The lesion may be ill defined, echopoor and other of complex focal lesions, some of which show increase reflectivity. Spleen is moderately enlarged. It may be associated with distortion of normal contour of spleen (Figs 10.17 and 10.18).

11

Urinary System

Kidneys

Physiology

The kidneys are the body's master chemists. They, not the intestinal tract, are the main waste disposal system. Blood passes through them continually and the kidneys leans and filter it ridding it of potentially dangerous waste. They help the production of red blood cells (RBCs) control the amount of potassium, sodium chloride, and other substances in the blood. The very smallest deviation, too much or too little, in the substances can be lethal. The kidneys also monitor and control vital water balance. Too much, and cells would drown; too little and they would dry up. In addition, the kidneys also see that the blood does not become too acid or alkaline.

Weighing approximately 5 oz each, the kidneys contain over a million tiny filtering units—*nephrons*. The curled and twisted end of each nephron is called a tubule. Twice each hour, the total body blood volume is filtered by these structures to prevent loss of valuable cells and essential blood proteins through the urine. The tubules also reabsorb 99% of the fluid process, returning just the right amount of essential vitamins, amino acids, glucose, hormones, etc. and is guarding to the urine any excesses.

Too much salt would result in an accumulation of fluid in blood and intercellular spaces. Face, feet and abdomen would puff up and eventually the heart unable to continue pumping against the growing load of gallons of retained fluid, would falter and stop. Too much sugar could mimic diabetes. Too much potassium (derived mainly from meat and fruit juices) would halt the heart. Too little potassium would also result in muscular failure especially of the breathing muscles.

The largest waste product is urea, the end product of protein digestion. Too little urea spells liver damage-too much uremic poisoning sets in as the name implies urea means too much urine in the blood, and this can lead to shock, coma, and death with the body coated with whitish crystals of urea (frost).

Everyday each kidney produces approximately one quart of urine. Microscopic droplets of urine pass out of each of the million tubules and feed into a tiny reservoir at the center of the kidneys. This connects with the bladder and the bladder with the outside. Wavelike muscular action occurs every 10–30 seconds pushing the fluid along the exit tubes. At night time, kidney activity slows to about 1/3rd of the daytime level.

Kidney production can be stepped up by a number of external causes for example body is chilled, anger, alcohol, caffeine, etc.

As the body ages, the kidneys become candidates for many ills. Floating kidneys would be a good example. Normally, kidneys rest in a bed of fat (*perinephric fat*) when the very obese reduce, much of this fat bed disappears, causing the tissues that anchor the kidneys to stretch and allowing the kidneys to begin to drift.

Kidney stones also increase as the body ages. They may occur when urine is too concentrated. Calcium salts, and uric acid simply crystalize out. Kidney stones may be tiny the size of gravel and pass to the outside without any awareness on the part of the body. If they grow larger to the size of pea the story is quite different. A kidney stone of this size as it attempts to pass through the exquisitely sensitive ureter (the tube leading to the bladder) can produce intense pain. In extreme cases, kidney stones may grow to be the size of a large grapefruit. A kidney stone of this size would require surgery.

Even when large numbers of nephrons have been destroyed, the kidneys can maintain function because of the large reserve capacity even if 90% of the nephrons stopped functioning, wise medical and dietary management can still provide years of life. This would mean keeping an ever vigilant eye on salt, potassium, and other substances in the food in an effort to achieve an exact balance. Any fluid intake must be exactly balanced with losses via the lungs, perspiration, urine. There are drugs too that now help in situations ones consider hopeless.

Remarkable laboratory tests are available to determine the exact nature of kidney problems. The basic test of course is urinalysis. Urinalysis can determine the presence of large quantities of protein which indicate that the filters are letting it escape from the blood.

If the tubules are inflamed solid matter such as cells, fats, proteins, solidify to the exact shape of the tubules and from time to time these substances which now coat the tubules are flushed out by the urine.

Analysis of the blood is also helpful in the diagnosis of kidney disease. The presence of excess urea in the blood would indicate that the kidneys are failing to rid the body of protein waste.

To promote proper and continued kidney functioning it is essential that one watches weight and blood pressure. Exercise, but not violent exercise, is helpful. Overworked muscles produce excess lactic acid, placing a burden on the kidneys. Extra fluid intake during the day is also helpful. Most people drink too little fluid. If urine becomes cloudy, smoky, or mahogany colored, medical attention should be sought immediately. Facial edema, nausea, blurred vision and weariness are common symptoms of an ailing kidney.

Anatomy

The kidney resembles a bean in shape. Average size of a kidney is approximately 8-9 cm in length and 4-6 cm in width and 2-4 cm in thickness. Usually, the left kidney is slightly larger than the right. The right kidney is generally lower than the left kidney, due to its displacement inferiorly by the liver. The kidneys lie behind the parietal peritoneum and because of this location being the membrane lining of the abdominal cavity kidneys are not considered as being in the abdominal cavity. They lie against the posterior wall of the abdomen, at the level of the last thoracic and first three lumbar vertebrae, or just above the waistline. A heavy cushion of fat normally keeps the kidneys up in position (*perinephric fat*) but vary from patient to patient so that thin individuals may suffer from ptosis (dropping) or one or both of these organs. Connective tissue (*renal fascia*) anchors both kidneys to surrounding structures and helps maintain them in normal position.

The medial surface of each kidney presents a concave notch called the *hilum*. Structures enter the kidneys through this notch. A tough, white fibrous capsule encases each kidney.

When a coronal section is made through a kidney, two kinds of substances are seen composing its interior: an outer layer, the cortex, and an inner portion, the *medulla*. The latter is divided into a dozen or more triangular wedges, the renal pyramids, the bases of which face the cortex and the apices, or renal papillae, the center of the kidney. The pyramids have a striated appearance as contrasted with the smooth texture of the cortical substance. The cortex extends onwards between each of the pyramids forming the renal columns.

Microscopically the kidneys are composed of peculiarly shaped structures resembling tiny funnels with proportionately long, convoluted stems. The upper portions of these anatomical funnels are called *Bowman's capsules*. Each capsule contains a cluster of capillaries designated as a glomerulus. A Bowman's capsule and its partially encased *glomerulus* are named a *renal corpuscle* or (*malpighian corpuscle*). Extending from each Bowman's capsule is a tubule composed of a convoluted portion, a loop of Henle, and straight or collecting tubules which give its characteristic striated appearance. A renal corpuscle, convoluted tubule, loop of Henle, and straight (collecting) tubule together constitute a uriniferous tubule or nephron, the physiological unit of the kidney. Of these, the renal corpuscle and convoluted tubule functions

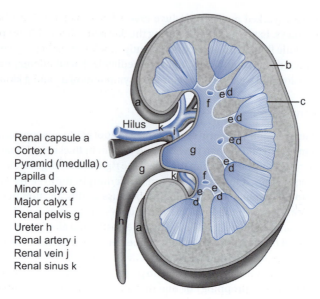

Renal capsule a
Cortex b
Pyramid (medulla) c
Papilla d
Minor calyx e
Major calyx f
Renal pelvis g
Ureter h
Renal artery i
Renal vein j
Renal sinus k

Fig. 11.1 Kidney-coronal section

as active structures in the formation of urine, while the straight or collecting tubules as their name indicates, serve merely as tubes for collecting the urine after it is formed.

Finally the urine is collected in a funnel-shaped structure called the pelvis (calyces) of the kidney, to be emptied into an epithelial-lined tube called a ureter (Figs 11.1 and 11.2).

Ureters

The two ureters are tubes from 20–24 cm long and are less than 0.5 cm in diameter. They lie behind the parietal peritoneum and extend from the kidneys to the posterior surface of the bladder. As the upper end of each ureter enters the kidney, it enlarges into a funnel-shaped basin named the *renal pelvis*. The pelvis expands into several branches called the *calyces*. Each calyx contains renal papillae. Urine is excreted into the calyces, then into the pelvis, and down the ureters into the bladder. The walls of the ureters are composed of three coats: a lining coat of mucous membrane, a middle coat of two layers of smooth muscle, and an outer fibrous coat. Valves guard the openings of the ureter into the urinary bladder. The ureters, together with their expanded upper portions, the pelvis and calyces, collect the urine as it forms and drain

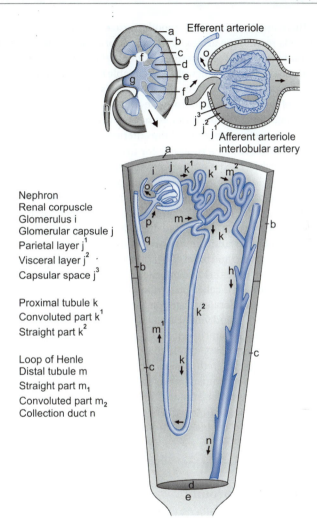

Fig. 11.2 Uriniferous tubules

it into the bladder. *Peristaltic waves* (about 1–5 per minute) force the urine down the ureters into the bladder.

Bladder

The bladder is a collapsible bag located directly behind the symphysis pubis. It lies below the parietal peritoneum which is deflected over its superior surface. There are three layers of smooth muscle which comprise its walls, while mucous membrane arranged in *rugae*, forms its lining. The parietal peritoneum covers only the superior bladder surface. Because of the rugae and the elasticity of the bladder walls, it is capable of considerable distention, although its capacity varies greatly with individuals. There are three openings in the floor of the bladder—two from the ureters, one into the urethra. The ureter openings lie at the posterior comers of the triangular shaped floor (*trigon*) and the urethral opening, at the anterior comer.

The bladder serves as a reservoir for urine before it leaves the body. Aided by the urethra, it expels urine from the body. Emptying of the bladder (*micturition*), *urination* or *voiding* is a reflex act of the first level when it is involuntary as in babes; of the third level, when it is involuntary. The normal stimulus for this reflex is pressure on the sensory receptors in the bladder *mucosa*. Voluntary control of micturition is possible only if the nerves supplying the bladder and urethra are all intact. Injury to these nerves (projection tracts of cord and brain and motor area of the cerebrum) or parts of this nervous system results in involuntary emptying of the bladder at intervals. Involuntary micturition is called *incontinence*. In the average bladder, 250 cc of urine will cause a moderately distended sensation and therefore the desire to void. Occasionally, an individual is unable to void even though the bladder contains an excessive amount of urine. This condition is known as *retention*. It often follows pelvic operations and childbirth. *Catheterization* (introduction of a rubber tube through the urethra into the bladder to remove urine) is used to relieve the discomfort accompanying retention. A more serious complication which is also characterized by the inability to void is called *suppression*. In this condition, the patient cannot void because the kidneys are not secreting any urine and therefore, the bladder is empty.

Kidneys Ultrasonography

Indications for Ultrasound

- Mass on IVP (in infants-palpable mass)
- Perirenal mass
- Nonvisualizing kidney on IVP
- Severe renal failure
- Renal transplant.

Anatomy

Parenchyma: Made up of glomeruli and tubules: nephrogram on IVP.

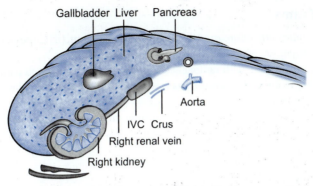

Fig. 11.3 Normal renal vascular anatomy (Transverse section)—
IVC and right renal vein
Abbreviation: IVC, inferior vena cava

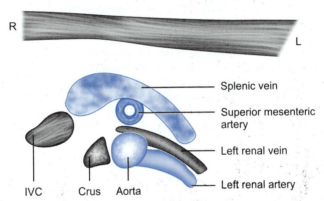

Fig. 11.4 Normal renal vascular anatomy (Transverse section)—
aorta and left renal vein
Abbreviation: R, right; L, left; IVC, inferior vena cava

Calyces: Where urine collects; portion of kidney seen containing contrast of IVP.

Pelvis: Area on medial aspect of kidney into which calyces empty.

Hilum: Medial aspect of kidney where artery and vein enter (Figs 11.3 and 11.4).

Laboratory Tests

Blood urea nitrogen (BUN) and creatinine-measure of substances are excreted by kidney measure of renal function.

X-ray Exams

- *IVP-contraindications are:* (i) allergy to contrast agent, (ii) kidney will not visualize in severe renal failure.
- Renal scan-done with radioactive isotope. Can be used when patient is allergic to contrast agents. If mass is present, will not differentiate solid from cystic mass.
- Retrograde pyelogram-requires instrumentation. Also cannot be done if patient is allergic to contrast. Done commonly in renal failure to rule out kidney obstruction as cause of etiology.
- Arteriography
- Nephrotomography
- Cyst puncture.

Diseases of the Kidney

Congenital Anomalies

Congenital anomalies of the kidneys are not uncommon. Occasionally there is fusion of the two, forming what is called a horseshoe kidney. One kidney may be small and deformed and often nonfunctioning. Abnormal vessels to the kidney may kink the ureter. Not in frequently, there may be a double ureter or congenital stricture of the ureter. Kidneys in unusual positions are frequently mistaken for tumors (Figs 11.5 to 11.8).

Trauma

Various types of crushing injuries of the loin may injure the kidney producing tears in its structure. The appearance of blood in the urine (Hematuria) following an injury to the loin is highly suggestive of an injury to the kidney. When the kidney is injured sufficiently to cause hemorrhage of considerable amount, operation may be necessary.

Renal Abscess

A hematogenous infection characterized by fever and dull pain in the region of the kidney.

Perinephric Abscess

An abscess in the fatty tissue is above the kidney which may arise secondary to an infection of the kidney or as a hematogenous infection originating in foci elsewhere in the body.

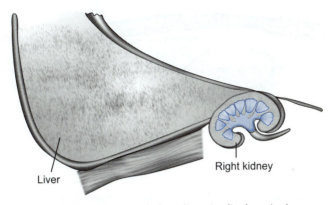

Fig. 11.5 Low lying kidney (Longitudinal section)

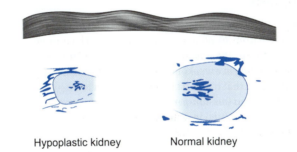

Hypoplastic kidney   Normal kidney

Fig. 11.6 Hypoplastic kidney (Transverse section)

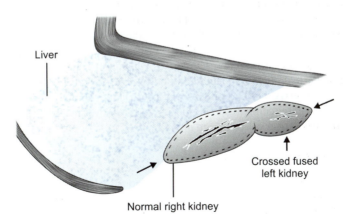

Fig. 11.7 Renal ectopia (Longitudinal section) (crossed fused)

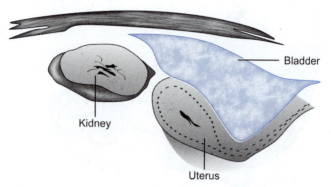

Fig. 11.8 Renal ectopia (Pelvic kidney) (Longitudinal section)

Nephroptosis

Commonly called "movable" kidney, is a condition found chiefly in thin, long waisted women from 30–50 years of age. The pad of fat normally surrounding the kidney is absent. The posture is usually poor and the abdominal muscles are relaxed, resulting in a weakness and dragging pain in the loin. At times the kidney may sag so that it almost reaches the pelvis when the patient stands (floating kidney) and this abnormal movability may produce torsion or kinks in the ureter accompanied by acute pain, nausea and vomiting and at times this obstruction of the ureter may result in fever and chills.

Hydronephrosis

Obstruction of the normal flow of urine will produce a damning up of urine with resultant back pressure on the kidney. If the obstruction is in the urethra or bladder, the back pressure affects both kidneys, but if the obstruction is in the ureter, due to stone or kink, only one kidney is damaged. When the obstruction is of long duration, it produces a dilatation of the ureter above the obstruction hydroureter, and the kidney becomes a mere shell filled with fluid. This condition is called hydronephrosis. If both kidneys are so diseased, their function of eliminating waste products from the body is markedly impaired and there is danger of death from *uremia*.

Urinary Calculi (Stones)

Stones are formed in the urinary tract due to deposits of crystalline substances secreted in the urine. They may be found anywhere from the kidney to the bladder and vary in size from mere granular deposits, called sand or gravel, to stones as large as an orange found in the bladder. Obviously, the resolution

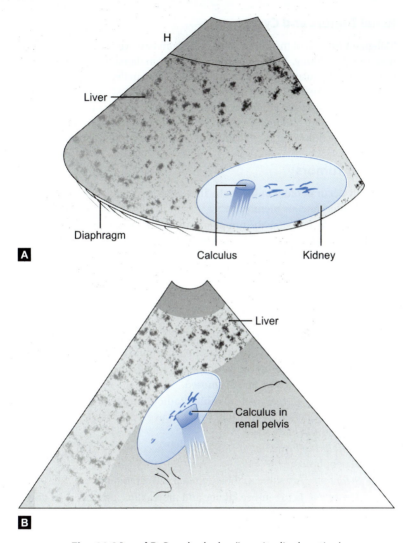

Figs 11.9A and B Renal calculus (Longitudinal section)
Abbreviation: H, head side

limits of present day ultrasonic equipment and the tissue surrounding the calculus will determine the possibility of ultrasonic detection. When the stones block the flow of urine, hydronephrosis develops, and the constant irritation of the stone may be followed by a secondary infection causing pyelitis, cystitis, etc. (Figs 11.9A and B).

Renal Tumors and Cysts

Malignant tumors of the kidney may arise from embryonal nests of adrenal tissue in the kidney, hypernephroma, or from malignant degeneration of renal tissue. The usual symptoms are hematuria. Usually, malignant disease of the kidney takes the form of *sarcoma* or carcinoma. Cysts of the kidney may be multiple, polycystic kidney or single. Polycystic kidney disease (PKD) is usually congenital and involves both kidneys; therefore, it is treated only by surgery if infection occurs within the cysts; solitary cysts often attain large size.

Bladder Tumors

Generally occur in older individuals. They arise as a cauliflower like growth in the bladder mucous membrane.

Bleeding occurs when the tumor is traumatized by the contraction of the bladder in urination. Obviously ultrasonic detection of bladder tumor must be carried out with a full bladder.

Renal Masses

Primary Neoplasms of the Kidney

- *Renal cell carcinoma (hypernephroma):* Accounts for 80% of primary neoplasms of the kidney. Two times more common in males than females.
  - *Symptoms and signs:* Hematuria, pain, palpable mass fever. 37% have metastatic disease when diagnosed.
  - *Treatment:* Surgery—if possible. Radiotherapy—if not able to do surgery. Chemotherapy—not very effective. Prognosis 5 year survival is 30–50% in early stages.
- *Transitional cell carcinoma (Rare tumor):* Accounts for 15% of primary renal neoplasms.
  - *Symptoms:* Are same as those in renal cell carcinoma.
  - *Treatment:* Is to remove kidney and ureter since this can seed down the ureter. 5 year survival rate is 47%.
- *Wilms' tumors (Childhood tumor):* 75% are seen before the age of five years. Bilateral tumors in 7%. No sex predilection.
  - *Symptoms:* Mass in 50%, hematuria in 20%, pain in 30% and elevated blood pressure in 75%.
  - *Treatment:* Nephrectomy followed by radiation therapy to the area of the kidney. Chemotherapy used also.
  - *Prognosis:* If tumor discovered in child less than 2 years of age, the two year survival is 73%.

Cystic Lesions of the Kidney

- Benign simple cyst usually an incidental finding. Usually cause no problems but must prove it is cyst rather than a neoplasm. Also must show walls of cyst to rule out tumor in wall of cyst or cystic changes within tumor.
- *Multicystic kidney disease:* 80% of cases are in children. Incidental findings are in adults. Children present with palpable mass. Adults are discovered when they are found to have a nonfunctioning kidney on intravenous pyelogram (IVP). The ureter will be either atretic or absent. Opposite kidney may hypertrophy.
- *Polycystic kidney disease:*
  - *Infantile type:* Seen in newborn. Bilateral. Not compatible with prolonged survival. Autosomal recessive inheritance. Presents with bilateral abdominal masses. Poor kidney function on IVP has liver cysts also.
  - *Adult type:* Age 40–50 when diagnosis made. Seen in 1:351 autopsies. Bilateral but one kidney may be more severe than the other. Autosomal dominant inheritance. Liver cysts seen in 1/3rd cases.
  - *Renal hemorrhage:* Seen after trauma. Patients on anticoagulants (Coumadin, Heparin) may bleed spontaneously into the kidney. May have hematuria, drop in hematocrit, pain.
  - *Renal abscess:* Usually results from spread of infection via blood (hematogenous). Will see local enlargement of kidney and calyceal distortion on IVP. Patient presents with fever, signs of kidney infection, elevated white blood cell count, pain (Fig. 11.10).

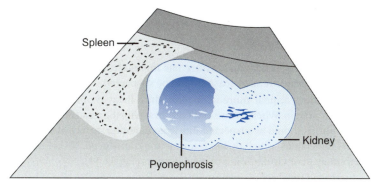

Fig. 11.10 Pyonephrosis (Longitudinal section)

Perirenal Masses

Retroperitoneal areas are relatively avascular so arteriography does not offer much diagnostically. Main means of detection is by displacement of other organs, i.e. kidney displaced on IVP, displacement of stomach and small bowel on UGI.

- *Sarcoma:* Solid tumor. May originate in retroperitoneal area but may invade kidney.
- *Neuroblastoma:* Accounts for 8–10% of childhood tumors. Solid tumor. 60% occur in retroperitoneum while 40% originate in adrenal.
    - *Symptoms:* Mass, elevated blood pressure. Elevated VMA.
    - *X-ray findings:* 50% have calcium. See mass which displaces kidney (Remember that Wilms' tumors involve the kidney whereas neuroblastomas displace kidney).
    - *Treatment:* Surgery, radiotherapy, chemotherapy.
- *Unilateral nonvisualizing kidney*
- *Bilateral nonvisualizing kidneys:* Must find etiology of renal failure. If failure is due to obstruction, may be possible to relieve obstruction and restore renal function. If end-stage, small scarred kidney is shown, then it is not a treatable lesion and must resort to dialysis and/or transplantation.
- *Renal transplants:* Usual site of implantation of the kidney is the iliac fossa.
- *Rejection of kidney:* Patient develops elevated blood pressure and other signs of renal failure.
- *Perirenal collection of fluid:* May compress kidney so that it does not function properly. This collection needs to be drained, urinomas, hematomas, lymphoceles. Due to compression, this mass mimic rejection crisis.

Chronic Renal Disease

When the renal parenchymal texture has increased echo amplitude. The diagnosis of chronic renal disease should be suspected.

The kidneys appear more echogenic than liver, smaller in sizes and irregular in margin. When there is difficulty in seeing the renal border, chronic pyelonephritis should be suspected. The irregular outer surface of the kidneys scatters the echoes, which do not return to the transduced. Therefore, there is extremely poor visualization of renal borders (Fig. 11.11).

Increased renal echogenicity with normal or increased in size of kidneys could be seen in severe amyloidosis or drug abuse (long standing heroin abuse) (Fig. 11.12).

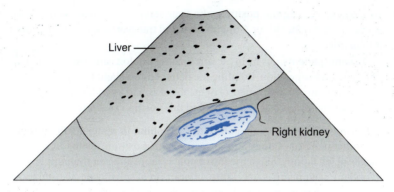

Fig. 11.11 Chronic pyelonephritis (Longitudinal section)

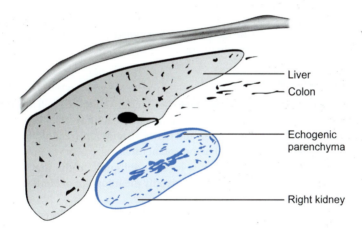

Fig. 11.12 Chronic renal disease (Longitudinal section) (Amyloidosis)

The surrounding retroperitoneal fat causes increased echogenicity which helps in diagnosing the position of kidneys in chronic renal disease.

Kidneys

Technique

No patient preparation is necessary. However, a well hydrated state is sometimes helpful. The transducer of highest frequency preferably 3.5 MHz should be used.

Right kidney: In supine position, the liver serves as acoustic window for examining the right kidney. Longitudinal and transverse scans are obtained at 1 cm intervals.

In some patients, gas from hepatic flexure of colon can obscure the right kidney in supine position. Rotating the patient into a slight LPO position will allow utilization of lateral aspect of right lobe of liver as a window. Longitudinal and transverse scans can be obtained in this position as discussed above.

Left kidney: It is best evaluated with the patient in a steep RPO or right decubitus position. Longitudinal scan in this position results in coronal images of left kidney. Since the lower pole is more anterior than upper pole an oblique scan plane is necessary. Inferior tip of spleen can be used as an acoustic window to visualize the upper pole of left kidney.

Transverse scans should be obtained perpendicular to oblique longitudinal scanning plane. It is best to study the kidneys in suspended deep inspiration.

Both the kidneys can be seen in prone positions as well. Longitudinal and transverse scans should be obtained.

Renal Transplant

Most renal transplants are located near the anterior abdominal wall in either the right or left iliac fossa. The standard longitudinal transverse planes are obtained of entire lower abdomen and pelvis. In addition, longitudinal and transverse images are obtained of transplant itself.

Since the transplant kidney is located obliquely in the iliac fossa, transverse scans are obtained first to identify the midpoint of kidney. Then longitudinal scan is taken.

Since it is important that any abnormal fluid collection be discerned from urinary bladder pre and postvoid scans are usually obtained.

Degree of hydration can be important particularly in attempting to identify mild degree of urinary tract obstruction.

Ultrasonic Renal Pelvicalyceal Echo

The introduction of gray-scale imaging has improved the assessment of renal abnormalities by allowing better detection and depiction of low-level echoes originating in the parenchyma and the hilar regions of the kidney. These echoes form the pelvicalyceal echo complex which in the normal kidney, appears as a filled cylindrical core of strong echoes seen in the medullary hilar portion of the kidney. Characteristic changes in the pelvicalyceal echo complex are seen with both parenchymal lesions and obstructive uropathy.

Normal Pelvicalyceal Echo Complex and Variants

The renal pelvicalyceal echo complex originates from the medullary hilar structures consisting of the individual calyces, infundibula, hilar vessels, and renal pelvis. When a slightly oblique longitudinal section is obtained through the medullary portion of the kidney, the entire length of the pelvicalyceal echo complex may be seen occupying the central two-thirds to three-fourths of the kidney. It is surrounded by a symmetrical rim of parenchyma. On transverse views, a cross-section of the cylinder is seen which appears as a relatively homogenous core of echoes located in the anterior medial portion of the "C shaped" renal parenchyma. Close analysis reveals small projections at the periphery of the pelvicalyceal echo complex which represent echoes originating from individual calyces. Using a high frequency transducer, a narrow sonolucent area may be seen within the pelvicalyceal echo complex in the normal kidney. This should not be confused with mild hydronephrosis. The sonolucent area represents the normal fluid-filled pelvis. Its size varies with the degree of distention of the renal pelvis. When a bifid renal pelvis or double collecting system is present, the pelvicalyceal echo complex will be split into two portions. Acoustic shadowing from overlying ribs may create a technical artifact similar of a bifid pelvis; the shadow from the offending rib can be readily identified because it will prevent both the renal outline and the central echo complex from being visualized.

Changes due to Hydronephrosis

The distended collecting system can be appreciated to a better extent as a sharply defined sonolucent collection within the echo-filled pelvicalyceal complex. The particular pattern of sonolucency within the pelvicalyceal echo complex varies in size and degree with the individual anatomy of the collecting system and the severity, duration, and location of the obstruction.

Enlargement of the renal pelvis due to minimal hydronephrosis cannot be reliably differentiated on the sonogram from the medially situated sonolucent collection seen with a normal fluid-filled extrarenal pelvis unless a previous study is available. With moderate hydronephrosis, three possible patterns of sonolucency develop. A continuous broad sonolucent band is seen with distension of the intrarenal pelvis. Oval sonolucent collections along the periphery of the central echo complex are seen when enlargement of the calyces occurs to a greater extent than enlargement of the renal pelvis. A mixed pattern is seen with enlargement of the pelvis and calyces. The sonographic findings of moderate hydronephrosis are particularly useful in the assessment of patients who have had a renal transplant or in patients with chronic renal failure in whom an IVP is technically difficult. In patients with renal transplants, the kidney is located so superficially that it has been possible to visualize the dilated infundibulum and calyces (Figs 11.13 to 11.15).

In severe chronic hydronephrosis, three different sonolucent patterns are seen within the pelvicalyceal echo complex. The "blown out sac" pattern is evidenced by a large, rounded sonolucent collection replacing the pelvicalyceal echo complex.

This pattern is caused by incorporation of the enlarged calyceal structures into the markedly distended pelvis. The "septated" pattern consists of large septated sonolucent collections representing markedly distended individual calyces. In hydrocalycosis, a congenital anomaly, a "pure" septated pattern may be seen due to markedly enlarged, ballooned calyces. The third pattern has a "dumbbell" configuration and is due to a ureteropelvic obstruction with marked enlargement of both the extrarenal pelvis and an intrarenal infundibulum. In between patterns maybe seen (Fig. 11.16).

Replacement of the pelvicalyceal echo complex by one of these patterns is reliable evidence of moderate or severe hydronephrosis. A peripelvic cyst may be mistaken for an extrarenal pelvis or minimal hydronephrosis, may be made by careful scanning in the transverse planes; an extrarenal pelvis or minimal hydronephrosis shows unequivocal evidence of communication between the eccentric, sonolucent collection and the pelvicalyceal echo complex.

A pattern simulating hydronephrosis may be seen in fibrolipomatosis. Relatively circular sonolucent collections may be seen but these contain low-level echoes. Pyonephrosis cannot be diagnosed unless the pus is thick enough to alter the sonolucency and through transmission characteristic of the enlarged collecting system. With thick, viscous pus, groups of echoes within the sonolucent pelvicalyceal echo complex may be seen.

Changes due to Cysts and Cystic Disease

Renal parenchymal cysts less than 1.5 cm in size may not be detected by sonography. A cyst produces deformity of the pelvicalyceal echo complex if it impinges on the medullary portion of the kidney. A simple renal cyst results in a characteristic smooth, sharply defined crescentic deformity of the adjacent pelvicalyceal echo complex. Scalloping of the margin of the pelvicalyceal echo complex is seen when multiple, simple renal cysts are present. Gross deformity of the entire pelvicalyceal echo complex is seen in moderate polycystic kidney disease. This should not be confused with hydronephrosis. A correct diagnosis of polycystic kidney disease is made through (a) the variability in the size of the cysts (b) the ragged walls of many of the cysts and (c) some echoes from the pelvicalyceal echo complex, which will be seen in spite of the distortion by the cysts unless there is concurrent hydronephrosis. In patients with

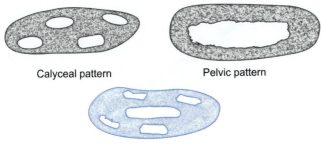

Calyceal pattern   Pelvic pattern

Mixed pattern

Fig. 11.13 Three sonolucent patterns that may be seen with moderate hydronephrosis

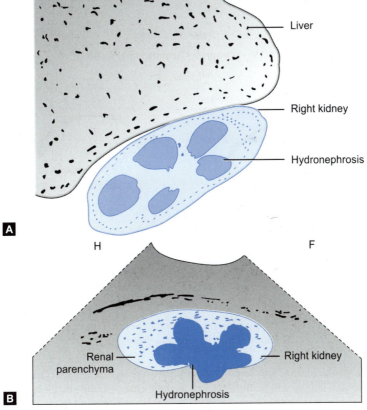

Figs 11.14A and B Hydronephrosis (Longitudinal section)
Abbreviations: H, head side, F, foot side

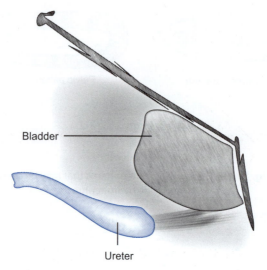

Bladder

Ureter

Fig. 11.15 Hydroureter (Longitudinal section)

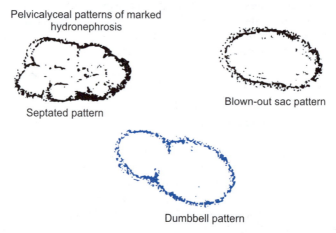

Pelvicalyceal patterns of marked hydronephrosis

Septated pattern

Blown-out sac pattern

Dumbbell pattern

Fig. 11.16 Different patterns of sonolucency that may be seen with long standing severe hydronephrosis

hydronephrosis in whom severe pyelonephritis has occurred, distinction from polycystic kidney will be difficult, but in the former, careful sectioning will reveal communications between the enlarged renal pelvis and the intrarenal sonolucent collections (Fig. 11.17).

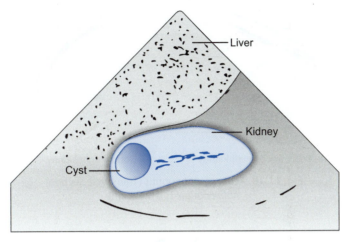

Fig. 11.17 Renal cyst (Longitudinal section)

In infantile polycystic kidney disease, the pelvicalyceal echo complex as well as the kidney is diffusely enlarged. Multiple small, cystic area representing the ectatic tubules are seen in the region of the junction between the cortex and medulla. In multicystic kidney disease of the newborn, both the pelvicalyceal echo complex and the renal parenchyma of the affected kidney are replaced by varying-sized, smooth walled, sonolucent collections.

Changes due to Edema and Vascular Alteration

Significant edema appears to diminish the size and strength of the echoes from the pelvicalyceal echo complex. Although this may be seen with acute pyelonephritis, or more commonly, transplant rejection, the sensitivity and specificity of this finding is not known. The papillary area in some cases becomes much more sonolucent possibly representing localized papillary edema. A distinct pattern of alteration has not been established for renal artery occlusion, renal vein thrombosis, or acute tubular necrosis, although when the edema phase is present, a decreased pelvicalyceal echo complex may be anticipated (Figs 11.18 to 11.21).

Changes due to Neoplasia

A variety of changes may be seen with neoplastic processes in the kidney. A locally confined neoplastic process may produce abrupt amputation of the pelvicalyceal echo complex or a "V" shaped splitting of the pelvicalyceal echo complex. The latter is more common in transitional cell carcinoma originating

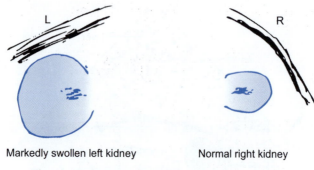

Markedly swollen left kidney   Normal right kidney

Fig. 11.18 Acute pyelonephritis (Transverse section)
Abbreviation: L, left; R, right

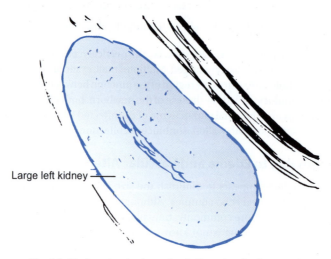

Large left kidney

Fig. 11.19 Renal vein thrombosis (Longitudinal section)

in the pelvis or calyx, but may also be seen with a polar hypernephroma involving the collecting system. A diffusely infiltrating hypernephroma may apparently diminish the increase of pelvicalyceal echo complex. Increase in size or absence of the pelvicalyceal echo complex is presumably determined by the degree of tumor replacement in the medullary hilar region, the extent of ventral necrosis and thrombosis (Figs 11.22 to 11.24).

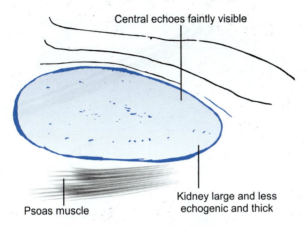

Fig. 11.20 Renal transplant-rejection (Longitudinal section)

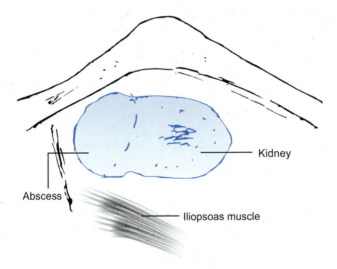

Fig. 11.21 Renal transplant-abscess (Transverse section)

Unilateral Large Kidney

- Compensatory hypertrophy due to disease or absence of other kidney.
- Cyst—Solitary
- Multicystic kidney
- Polycystic kidney

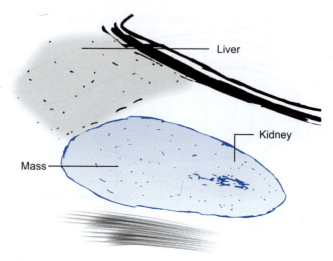

Fig. 11.22 Hypoechoic renal carcinoma (Longitudinal section)

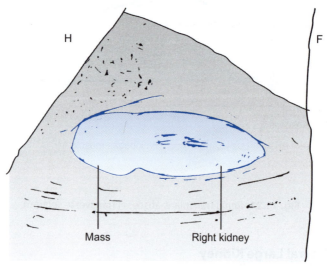

Fig. 11.23 Hyperechoic renal neoplasm (Longitudinal section)

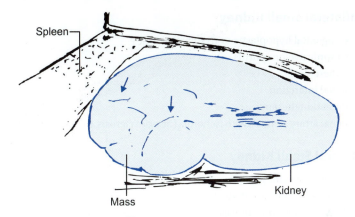

Fig. 11.24 Hypernephroma (Longitudinal section)

- Neoplasm
  - Hypernephroma
  - Wilms' tumor
  - Metastases
- Ureteric obstruction with hydronephrosis
- Renal vein thrombosis
- Trauma
- Transplant rejection (acute).

Bilateral Large Kidney

- Bilateral duplication
- Bilateral obstructive hydronephrosis
- Nephritis or nephrosis
  - Toxic nephrosis
  - Lipid nephrosis
  - Acute pyelonephritis
  - Acute glomerulonephritis.
- Polycystic disease (adult or infantile)
- Bilateral metastases
- Lymphoma.

Unilateral Small Kidney

- Congenital hypoplastic or dysplastic kidney
- Chronic pyelonephritis
- Tuberculosis
- Renal infarction
- Radiation therapy
- Renal artery stenosis with ischemia (arteriosclerosis, thromboembolism).

Bilateral Small Kidney

- Chronic pyelonephritis
- Chronic glomerulonephritis
- Arteriolar nephrosclerosis
- Ischemia (B/L renal artery stenosis)
- Senile atrophy
- Gouty nephritis.

Decrease Size of Part of Kidney

- Ischemic-infarct pyelonephritis
- Trauma
- Abscess (healed)
- Tuberculosis.

Unilateral Nonvisualization of Kidney on IVP

- Ectopic kidney
- Fractured kidney
- Neoplasm
- Obstruction of ureter
    - Calculus
    - Stricture
    - Neoplasm
- Renal artery obstruction
    - Stenosis
    - Trauma
- Absent kidney (congenital, postnephrectomy)
- Renal vein obstruction (thrombosis, tumor)
- Multicystic kidney
- Tuberculosis.

Localized Bulge of Renal Outline

- Cyst
- Localize hypertrophy (e.g. in pyelonephritis)
- Neoplasm
- Abscess
- Hematoma
- Hypertrophy of upper pole
- Normal
  - Dromedary hump
  - Fetal lobulation.

Urinary Bladder

Physiology

Undoubtedly the least glamorous organ in the human body, the bladder is a constant source of annoyance and embarrassment. Its urgings can interrupt sleep, important business conferences, and even peak emotional encounters. It does not ask for attention. It demands it.

While one might think of the intestines as the main waste disposal system this is an erroneous concept. The intestinal tract can go on strike for a week or in extreme cases or several weeks without grave danger to the body. But if the urinary system stops for more than few days it can spell real trouble.

Roughly the shape of a punching bag, bladder capacity varies with individuals from 6–24 oz. In the normal range capacity is about one pint. Day and night kidneys dribble urine into the bladder via two tiny ureters or tubes about the size of pencil lead and approximately 12 inches long.

The exit to the outside of the body is the pencil-size urethra. The amount of fluid emptied through this orifice varies tremendously-from one pint to two gallons per day. The average amount is being three pints. Volume is largely determined by fluid losses from the sweat glands and the lungs. When perspiration increases urine production falls. Fortunately urine production falls during sleep to about one quarter of the daytime level.

When the bladder empties, muscles at the top contract first, then those below add their squeeze. In effect the bladder wrings itself out. How often this is done is determined by many things. Worry, anxiety and fear hoist blood pressure and thereby stop up kidney activity and urine production. Mental stress, the excitement of a ball game or anger tends to tighten the muscular walls of the bladder. The bladder may not be full but may wish to be relieved just the same.

During pregnancy, the constant pressure of the weight of the fetus increases the urge to empty the bladder. On cold days, the frequency increases. To conserve heat, the bloodstream detours in blood vessels. More blood goes to internal organs. As kidneys filter more blood they produce more urine. Certain condiments also irritate the bladder, such as mustard, pepper and ginger along with tea and coffee. Alcohol is similarly irritating, particularly gin.

An examination of urine can reveal an enormous amount about what is happening elsewhere in the body. If urine is noted to be persistently colored, malodorous and discolored, medical help should be sought. If the urine is too deep an amber color, this may mean that the kidneys are doing too good a job of concentration, or it may mean only that the individual has been playing tennis and sweating so heavily that he has not a lot of fluid left for the kidneys to dispose of. If the urine is cloudy this may indicate kidney illness or it can be meaningless. Urine tends to cloud after heavy exercise. If there is blood in the urine this can be deadly serious. The presence of blood in the urine should prompt immediate medical attention.

Today, elaborate urine testing is a popular medical practice. The specific gravity of fluid—its weight in relation to a similar amount of pure water—can be very revealing. If it is too low the kidneys are doing a poor job of concentrating wastes; if it is too high, it may mean the patient is dehydrated. The presence of uric acid or high levels of uric acid may indicate stones or gouty kidneys. Also associated with elevated uric acid content in the urine are heart and kidney disease, psoriasis and endocrine disorders.

To some extent, virtually all organs empty waste or excess production in urine. This is particularly true of glands. With pregnancy for example, surplus female hormones pass out of the body in urine. Hence, the urine tests for pregnancy.

Urination is considerably more complex than simply emptying a bag of water. The bladder contains two valves called sphincters. One is at the base of the bladder and opens automatically when the bladder is distended. The second is a little lower and is under voluntary control. Opening of the first sphincter makes the body conscious of a desire to urinate. Opening of the second sets events in motion. Controlled opening of this second valve must be learned in early childhood. It is interesting to note that we come into this world as bedwetters, and at death, the body loses control of this restraining valve and we become bedwetters again.

Incontinence is general with the paralyzed and the aged. Neurogenic (paralyzed) bladder is another matter. This usually traces to congenital brain or spinal cord damage of some type.

To a large degree, the force of the urinary stream is a good measure of general health. An enlarged or diseased prostate in the male can reduce or cut off flow. Strictures traceable to venereal or other diseases—do the same. Tumors can also be involved.

While it may seem strange, the body can get along quite well without a bladder. If a devastating cancer required removal of the bladder, surgeons would simply hook the ureters from the kidney to the large intestine.

While the bladder is capable of reflecting troubles elsewhere in the body, it has its own particular set of ailments. Stones often form in the bladder. They can block both the entrance and exit tubes. This means exquisite pain. Urine backing up in kidneys long enough, can lead to uremic poisoning and death.

Bladder stones are composed of minerals precipitated out of urine that for one reason or another has become too concentrated. For some very complex reasons, stones are far more common in warm climates than in cooler area. Lack of exercise also seems to lead to the presence of stones. They vary in size. Some may be tiny bits of gravel that pass readily out of the bladder. In extreme cases, stones have grown to fourteen pounds in size.

Curiously stones, as large as oranges may be tolerated by the bladder for years, giving rise to no serious symptoms at all. As long as they do not have jagged edges to injure tissues, and so long as they do not block vital passages, the body can live with them, when stones do cause difficulties, they must be surgically removed. Or, the physician may pass a specially equipped cytoscope through the urethra. This small tube is equipped with lenses for observation and has nut cracker like jaws to crush stones to passable size.

The biggest, most common problem of the bladder is cystitis. Microbes creep into the bladder causing a very uncomfortable infection. At one time or another virtually all women experience this condition. The reason they are so much more prone to it than men is obvious. The female urethra is only an inch or two in length. The male tube passing through the penis is far longer, eight to twelve inches. Thus in women, microbes from the outside of the body have only a very short distance to travel to reach the bladder. Fortunately, cystitis is more of a nuisance than a deadly serious disease. It leads to frequent urination, burning and a general feeling of discomfort and can usually be corrected with antibiotics or sulfur drugs. For all the attention, the bladder demands, and all the troubles it can cause, one might expect it to rank high in importance among the body organs. However, this is not the case. In final analysis, the bladder is simply a cistern regularly filled-regularly drained. Nevertheless, it continues to boss the body as long as it is in existence.

Adrenal Ultrasonography

Adrenal Glands

The adrenal glands are two, flattened yellowish-bodies approximately 4 cm long which lie on the upper anatomical surface of the kidneys. They are also called *Suprarenal glands*.

They pour their secretions directly into the bloodstream, although they are ductless and are therefore endocrine glands. Their function is closely related to other ductless glands such as the thyroid, pituitary, liver and gonads in controlling the normal growth and development of the body in maintaining a certain equilibrium among its various processes. Each ductless gland, besides its specific function, seems to have an effect on every other ductless gland.

Each gland is composed of two distinct, separate layers, the yellowish cortex which covers the whole external surface and the gray central part, or medulla. The cells of the medulla secrete a substance called *epinephrine* or *adrenaline*, which acts as an emergency messenger to activate the sympathetic nervous system in times of emotional stress. Under the influence of emotions such as fear and anger the adrenals, stimulated by the sympathetic nerves mobilize body resources for such exertions as struggle or flight. The actual effect of this sudden spillage of epinephrine into the blood causes high blood pressure (BP) and pulse rate, inhibition of digestion, erection of the hair, dilatation of the pupil and rise in the blood sugar.

Roughly the shape of a tricorne hat, not much larger than the tip of a finger the adrenal gland weights about as much as a nickel. But its abilities are immense. It has the capacity of crippling, sickening or killing the patient. Absolutely essential to life, the removal of both glands would result in death in 1 or 2 days, unless supplementary artificial hormone therapy is initiated immediately. Under-activity results in weakness and debilitation. Over-activity cause premature sexual development and premature closure of bone ends.

Long a mystery organ, chemists were the ones who discovered the virtuosity of the adrenal glands, especially the cortisone like hormones it contained which could be used in treating hundreds of diseases from gout to asthma.

The architecture of the adrenal glands are that they have one of the richest networks of blood vessels in the entire body, and a large reserve capacity. Only 10% of tissue is required to maintain normal body needs.

The adrenals produce two sets of hormones. The medulla (or core) make one set; the cortex (or rind) the other. From the core exists the unique feature of a direct hotline to the brain. In the presence of any strong emotion—sudden rage or overwhelming fear—the medulla receives the information immediately. Not knowing the nature of the emergency, the adrenals prepare the body for both fight or flight. The medulla begins pouring two hormones adrenalin and nor adrenalin into the bloodstream.

Body response is extraordinary. The liver immediately releases stored sugar into the bloodstream providing instant energy. The hormones shut down skin blood vessels causing pallor, and shift this blood supply into muscles and internal organs. The heart speeds up, the arteries tighten to elevate BP, digestion halts and clotting time is quickened in case of injury.

All of these activities take place in seconds and the body is virtually super human in terms of surviving by running, jumping or hitting harder than *ever* before possible.

However these extreme functions cannot last indefinitely because the body would race itself to death. The same stresses that trigger adrenalin production also cause the hypothalamus to stimulate pituitary gland production of adrenocorticotropic hormone. This substance in turn targets the adrenal cortex to step up its production of hormones. Under stressful conditions these hormones act to maintain BP and blood flow to vital organs, helping convert fat and protein into sugar for immediately usable energy and soon everything is once again under control.

The hormones produced by the cortex fall into three categories:

1. Those from cortisone family supervise metabolism of fats, carbohydrates and protein.
2. Those which control water and mineral (electrolyte) balance in the body.
3. Sex hormones to supplement those produced by the gonads.

The hormones cannot be stored, therefore, they must be manufactured constantly and any excess destroyed by the liver.

Maintaining an exact balance is very important. Disease or injury knocking out the working cells of the cortex formerly was a death sentence. The symptoms weight and BP dropped; appetite dwindled; nausea; vomiting BP dropped; patient steadily grew weaker and weaker and usually death was welcomed. Now, in light of proper diagnosis, artificial hormones can be administered and life maintained.

Too much *cortisol* hormone can be as critical as too little. In this case, the arms and legs shrivel as the excess amount of hormone converts muscle protein into sugar. Drained of minerals bones become brittle. Fat accumulates across the back and in the fold of the abdomen, overloading the now spindly legs. Blood pressure soars and mental aberrations become common.

Another major hormone, *aldosterone*, is helpful in maintaining the mineral and water balance in the body. Too much aldosterone even a speak-spells trouble. Vital potassium is lost in the urine, excess *sodium* is retained. Muscles weaken and may become paralyzed. The BP and heart rate soar, fingers tingle, headaches are continuous and almost unbearable. Overproduction of aldosterone is usually caused by a tumor. Removal of the tumor results in cure.

Continuous excessive strain through worry, anger or fear should definitely be avoided.

Right Adrenal Gland

It is situated between the liver and crus of diaphragm, posterior to inferior vena cava (IVC) and just cephaloid to right kidney.

Retroperitoneal fat surrounds the adrenal gland.

The best scan plane for visualizing the right adrenal gland is through the intercostal space on a lateral aspect of abdomen (left lateral decubitus).

The right adrenal gland usually appears as a linear or curvilinear structure situated with in highly reflective retroperitoneal fat. The acoustic texture of adrenal gland is similar to that of crus of the diaphragm (Fig. 12.1).

Left Adrenal Gland

Left adrenal gland is a triangular structure usually situated anterior to the left kidney. A lateral posterior approach is most often successful in visualization of left adrenal gland. The proper scan plane lines up the left kidney and the aorta so that both can be visualized on the scan.

When this posterolateral approach lines up the kidney and aorta the transducer is turned 90° so that longitudinal plane of left adrenal gland may be obtained. The left adrenal gland is situated between the upper pole of left kidney and aorta with crus adjacent to the aorta (Fig. 12.2).

Adrenal Glands: Technique

Adrenal glands are located, near the upper poles of right and left kidneys and moves along with kidneys with respiration motion. It is performed with patient fasting. A 3.5 MHz medium focal zone transducer is usually appropriate. Adrenal masses 2 cm or larger can be readily identified sonographically.

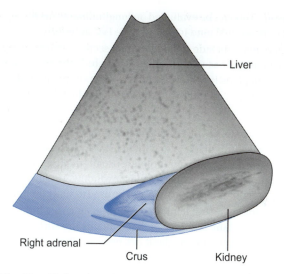

Fig. 12.1 Right adrenal gland (longitudinal coronal plane)

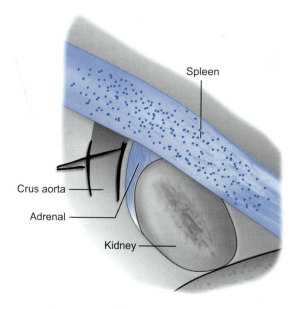

Fig. 12.2 Left adrenal gland (posterolateral approach)

Right adrenal: This can be evaluated on longitudinal scans through the IVC. Masses of right adrenal tend to displace the IVC anteriorly.

With patients right side up longitudinal sections using the right kidney and right lobe of liver as window are used to study the right adrenal gland. An oblique scan plane is achieved which contains upper pole of right kidney just posterior to IVC. The right adrenal gland lies between liver and crus of diaphragm.

Left adrenal: Masses of left adrenal gland can be frequently identified on transverse scans through left lateral intercostal spaces using the spleen as a window. Varying degree of inspirations are usually required to identify the left adrenal area through the intercostal acoustic window. Modification of coronal scans in both decubitus positions can also be used to study the adrenal glands.

With left side up, using left kidney and spleen as a window an oblique longitudinal scan plane is achieved that contains the aorta and upper pole of left kidney. The left adrenal gland lies between these two structures just lateral to the crus of diaphragm.

Ultrasound Appearances

Pseudocyst

It appears as rounded fluid filled area, usually have all the features of fluid mass (anechoic mass of smooth margin). These cysts are due to hemorrhage. In some cases, some clot may persist which may appear as solid projection in the cyst (Fig. 12.3).

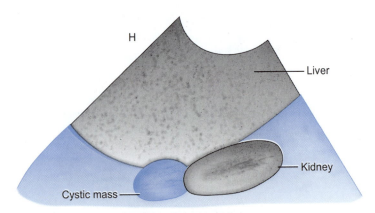

Fig. 12.3 Right adrenal mass (Longitudinal section) (pseudocyst-hemorrhage)
Abbreviation: H, head

Calcification of Adrenal Gland

Highly reflective borders and shadowing is seen (Fig. 12.4).

Pheochromocytoma

They are usually over 2 cm size. They cause localized elevation of IVC anteriorly and posteroinferior depression of right kidney. Drapping of right renal vein is seen anteriorly. Mass is usually of low level echoes (Figs 12.5 and 12.6).

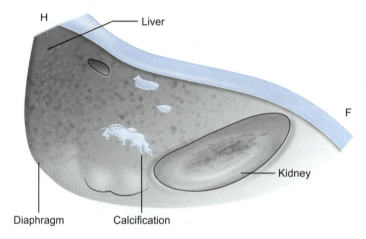

Fig. 12.4 Calcification of adrenal gland (Longitudinal section)
Abbreviations: H, head; F, foot

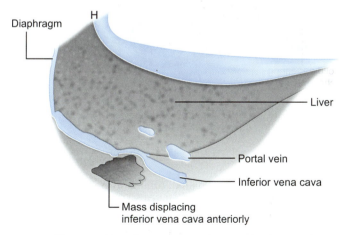

Fig. 12.5 Pheochromocytoma (Longitudinal section)
Abbreviation: H, head

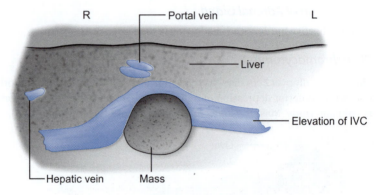

Fig. 12.6 Pheochromocytoma (Transverse section)
Abbreviation: R, right; L, left; IVC, inferior vena cava

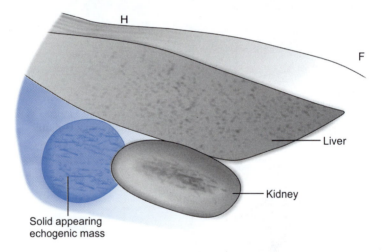

Fig. 12.7 Neuroblastoma (Longitudinal section)
Abbreviation: H, head; F, foot

Neuroblastoma

It is an adrenal malignancy of childhood. Tumors are frequently large. There is tendency toward microscopic calcification in neuroblastoma usually leads to a relatively solid appearing echogenic mass on ultrasound examination.

Usually, fat line (perirenal retroperitoneal fat line) is displaced anteriorly (Fig. 12.7).

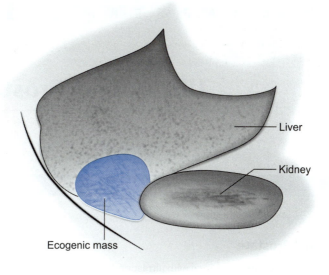

Fig. 12.8 Myelolipoma (Longitudinal section)

Myelolipoma

It is an uncommon tumor. The tumor is composed of varying amount of fat and bone marrow elements.

The mass appears to be echogenic (Fig. 12.8).

Ultrasound: Prostate

MALE PELVIS

Prostate

Normal Prostate

When the prostate is examined with ultrasound the urinary bladder should be filled. The transducer must be angled more caudally for both longitudinal and transverse scans. The prostate is situated quite caudally and if the transducer beam is perpendicular to the table top or slightly cephalad in angulation the prostate gland cannot be visualized.

Longitudinal Scan

The prostate appears as a soft echogenic region posterior to the urinary bladder and cauded to the seminal vesicles (Fig. 13.1).

Transverse Scan

With caudal angulation with the prostate indenting the posterior aspect of urinary bladder. In the center of the prostate gland a strong central echo represents the urethra and periurethral glands within the prostate (Fig. 13.2).

Benign Prostatic Hypertrophy

It is suggested when a markedly enlarged prostate without disruption of the prostatic capsule is present on ultrasound.

Longitudinal Scan

Circular appearance of prostate is seen. This is suggestive of enlargement of prostate (Fig. 13.3).

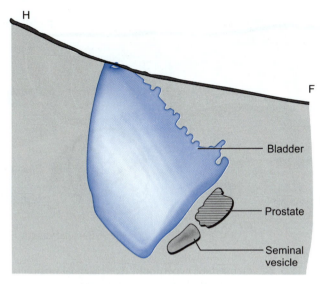

Fig. 13.1 Normal prostate (Longitudinal section)
Abbreviations: H, head end, F; foot end

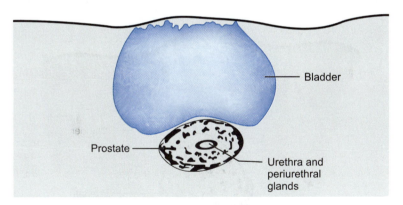

Fig. 13.2 Normal prostate (Transverse section)

Transverse Scan

Marked indentation to the posteroinferior urinary bladder wall caused by the enlarged prostate. Ultrasound demonstrates a nodularity to the prostate with two prominent curvilinear indentations on the posterior aspects of bladder wall (Fig. 13.4).

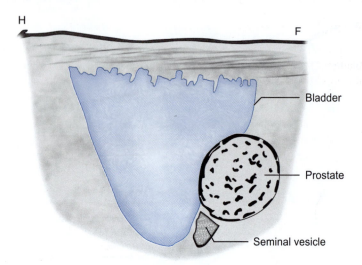

Fig. 13.3 Benign prostatic hypertrophy (Longitudinal section)
Abbreviations: H, head end, F; foot end

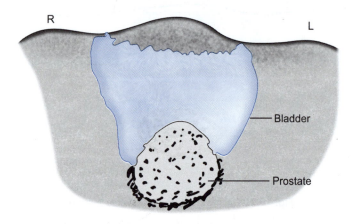

Fig. 13.4 Benign prostatic hypertrophy (Transverse section)
Abbreviation: R, right; L, left

Prostatic Carcinoma

The prostate is enlarged causing indentation to the posterior aspect of urinary bladder. Uneven echo pattern (irregular echogenicity) and irregular wall to the prostate are highly suggestive of prostatic carcinoma (Figs 13.5 and 13.6).

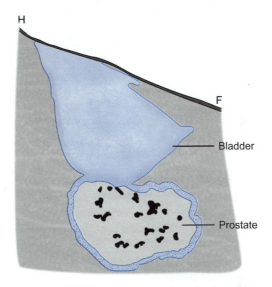

Fig. 13.5 Prostatic carcinoma (Longitudinal section)
Abbreviations: H, head end, F; foot end

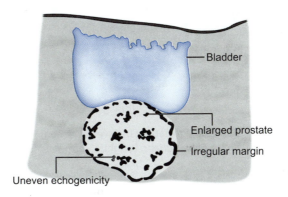

Fig. 13.6 Prostatic carcinoma (Transverse section)

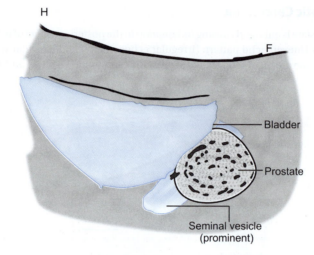

Fig. 13.7 Prostatitis (Longitudinal section)
Abbreviations: H, head end, F; foot end

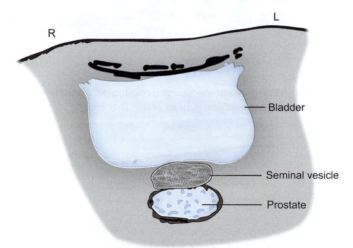

Fig. 13.8 Prostatitis (Transverse section)
Abbreviations: R, right; L, left

Prostatitis

The prostate has a fairly even echo pattern. The seminal vesicles, however, appear much more lucent and large as compared with normal findings (Figs 13.7 and 13.8).

Abdominal Sonography

Introduction

A discussion of abdominal sonography must be preceded by a review of the structures that not only support but divided the various body cavities or spaces.

The *peritoneum* is an often mentioned but perhaps not fully understood entity. It is a membranes composed of serous material which exists in two layers. Its purpose is to line the abdominal cavity and to cover the *viscera* which lies within it.

The lining portion of the peritoneum is called the *parietal peritoneum* and the opposing side of it which covers the organ is called the *visceral peritoneum*.

Another important structure in the abdominal cavity are the *ligaments* which not only connect bones but also exist as special folds of the peritoneum which pass between the organs and the abdominal wall and hold the viscera in place. These ligaments also serve the purpose simultaneously of transmitting blood vessels and nerves to and from these same organs.

The *omentum* is one such ligament which also can be discussed as having three major groups: (1) The *lesser omentum*, which is the ligament passing from the lesser curvature of the stomach and the first part of the duodenum to the inferior surface of the liver. The *hepatic artery*, *portal vein* and *main bile duct* are carried within its free margin; (2) The *greater omentum* which passes between the greater curvature of the stomach and the transverse colon and hangs down like an apron over the small intestine and finally; (3) A thin shaped fold of peritoneum called the mesentery, which enfolds most of the small intestine and anchors it to the posterior abdominal wall.

While some organs within the abdomen are not covered by peritoneum they lie posterior to the peritoneal cavity rather than within it and are called retroperitoneal organs. The *abdominal aorta*, *pancreas*, most of the *duodenum* and the *kidneys* are such organs.

Another organ we 'see' with ultrasound but disdain because of its poor sound transmitting abilities is the *stomach*, which lies in the upper part of the abdominal cavity just below the diaphragm.

The superior most part of the stomach houses an opening between the *esophagus* and the stomach called the *cardiac orifice*. The next portion of the stomach is called the fundus and the final two thirds of the organ is termed the body, while the distal portion of this is called the *pylorus*.

Whenever speaking of the stomach it is important to consider its two major areas the *anterior* and *posterior* aspects. The medial border of the stomach is called the *lesser curvature* and its lateral border is called the *greater curvature*.

Within the stomach an interesting phenomenon occurs.

Whenever the stomach is empty, the mucous membrane that lines it is thrown into longitudinal folds called *rugae*; when the stomach is full and stretches to contain food or liquids the rugae smooth out and disappear.

Gastric glands are situated in the fundus and body of the stomach and secrete digestive juices to aid in the preparation of food for the process of digestion.

As mentioned previously the stomach presents an ambivalent image to the sonographer. When filled with food and air it casts a tremendous shadow over organs of interest to the sonographer. However, when fluid-filled the stomach can be either a blessing or a pit-fall. Knowingly filling the stomach with fluid, the sonographer may attempt to use it as a window into the abdomen and the organs which lie below it. Unknowingly filled with fluid it may be mistakenly identified as a cystic mass such as a pancreatic pseudocyst.

Another inhabitant of the abdominal cavity that must be recognized and dealt with by circumvention is the intestines. The small intestine is about 21 feet long and one inch in diameter and extends from the pyloric opening of the stomach all the way down to the entrance of the large intestines. This coiled mass of air filled bowel can wreak havoc on the ultrasound examination. It is because of the area occupied by the intestine and the gas within it that we as sonographers try our best to see that the patient is properly prepared for the abdominal ultrasound study.

The small intestine can be divided into three main portions; the *duodenum, jejunum and ileum.*

The first few inches of small intestine is called the duodenum and is seen as a structure forming a C-shaped curve around the head of the pancreas. On the inner wall of the duodenum is a small elevation of tissue called the *duodenal papillae*. It is into this area that the *common bile duct* and the *pancreatic ducts* open. It is an area situated approximately 3 inches below the pylorus of the stomach. Most commonly these two ductal system will open side-by-side but separate from one another sharing only a thin common wall. Most of the duodenum is *retroperitoneal*.

The next portion, the jejunum, is about 8 feet in length with its final most distal portion, the ileum, measuring approximately 12 feet in length. Both of these parts are suspended from the posterior and abdominal walls by the mesentery.

While the sonographer's main concern involving the intestines is its sound-blocking contents (gas) occasionally the intestines or bowel, become fluid-filled and may present an unusual, cystic and honeycombed pattern. Sonographers beware, do not mistake this for a multiloculated cyst mass.

Gastrointestinal Ultrasound

Sonography using linear or curved sector scanner of 3.5 and 5 MHz is needed. Sonography is providing characteristic diagnostic clues in several diseases of gastrointestinal tract.

General Sonographic Findings

Peritoneal Cavity

Free fluid can be detected in following areas using a full bladder:
- In the pouch of Douglas, in the left or right lateral position
- In paracolic spaces
- Subphrenically on both sides or in hepatorenal recess.

Free fluid characteristically shift when patient position is changed.

Fecal contamination of peritoneal cavity is distinguished by flocky blotch particles swimming in fluid (Fig. 14.1). Presence of free air and feces together also suggests bowel perforation. This is also a reliable' evidence of anastomotic leakage.

Free Air

Characteristically appears as linear reverberation echoes.

Differential diagnosis of this finding includes intestinal gas which causes mussel-shaped, breath dependent column of air. Abscesses, hematomas and infiltration may also appear fluid like hypodense areas with internal echoes depending on the extent of organization. Hematoma normally gives a 'honey comb' appearance.

Sonographic detection of thickened gastrointestinal wall may be found in inflammatory, hemorrhagic and ischemic diseases and in benign or malignant tumors.

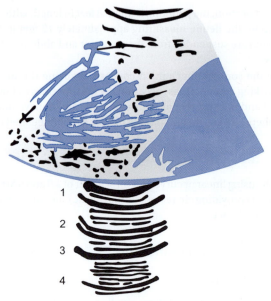

Fig. 14.1 Sonographic appearance of free fecal matter with typical snow flakes appearance in free fluid and free gases (Fg) with characteristic reverberation echoes in peritoneal cavity

Stomach Duodenum

Lutz describe the sonographic phenomenon of cockade, which occurs due to circular echo poor seromuscularis, surrounding a central echogenic mucosa and intraluminal contents. In healthy subject hypodense layer is 3 ± 1 mm in the stomach corpus in fasting state. When the stomach is distended with fluid the wall thickness decreases to 2.5 ± 1 mm.

We can visualize individual layers of gastric wall with 5 and 7.5 MHz scan. These make it possible to discern the depth of penetration and extent of inflammatory or tumorous changes of gastric and intestinal wall.

A pathological cockade, i.e. wall thickness exceeding the limits, was initially considered diagnostic of malignant gastric process (Fig. 14.2). Today we know that such changes can occur even with benign gastric and duodenal ulceration at any location.

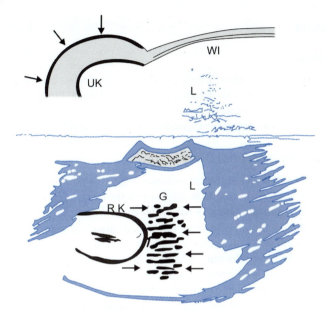

Fig. 14.2 Perforated duodenal ulcer
Abbreviations: G, free gases in the recessus hepatorenal is marked by arrows; L, liver; RK, right kidney; UK, pathological wall thickening (ulcer cockade); WI, normal gastric wall layers

Ulcer Perforation

In ulcer perforation following changes may serve as useful criteria:
- Pathological cockade
- Gastric distention caused by liquid retention
- Edema of the rest of the gastric wall
- Free feces and fluid
- Free anechoic fluid
- Air in peritoneal cavity (73%).

Pathological duodenal cockades are found occasionally in duodenal diverticula and in malignant tumors in the duodenal area.

Sonographically a swollen, fluid filled stomach, appearing like a balloon, is found in pyloric stenosis, atonic stomach in proximal intestinal obstruction.

Hypertrophic pyloric stenosis in early infancy has recognized to have, classical ultrasound features—'Pathological pyloric cockade.'

Intestine

Enteritis

Patient with mild diarrhea, intralumen fluid sequestration can be detected on sonography along with minimal anechoic peritoneal fluid. There is no uniform intestinal dilatation. Hyperperistalsis may result in quick changes in appearance which may be seen in real time observation.

Incomplete Intestinal Obstruction

Clinical diagnosis includes gastroenteritis, biliary or renal colic, history of abdominal surgery leading to suspicion of adhesion, intake of bulky food (mushroom, cabbage, beans, salads, whole meal bread).

Real-time sonography reveals fluid filled intestinal segments, dilated to up to 2.5 cm and with limited amplitude of contraction with hypodense wall edema (≥ 3 mm) the ratio of luminal diameter during contraction and relaxation is more important than absolute values. Often thick intraluminal bulk food products and free transudate fluid can also be visualized.

It is also possible to observe dilated and collapsed loops (hungry intestinal segments) lying side by side.

Peristaltic wall movements are animated, and intraluminal mobility of particles paradoxical.

Obstruction of Small and Large Intestine

Ileus stasis of luminal contents in the prestenotic intestinal segment is a major pathological phenomena of intestinal obstruction leads to progressive intestinal distention with massive proliferation of bacteria, formation of putrefactive gases hypoxic, endotoxin related damage of mucosa and edema of intestinal wall (Fig. 14.3).

Sonographically the approximate site of obstruction can be determined since typical features like kerckring's folds and haustrations are easily identifiable (Fig. 14.3). Differentiation between paralytic and persistent peristalsis can also be done.

Mesenteric Infarction

At the onset hyperactive peristalsis with rapidly increasing edema of intestinal wall and mesenteric edema measuring up to 10 mm can be seen sonographically; along with a radiological gasless abdomen. At the same time large amount of transudative fluid can be found.

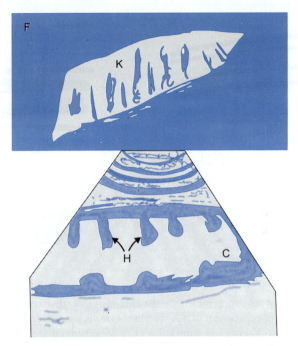

Fig. 14.3 Classic sonographic signs of small and large bowel obstruction by identification of mucous membrane structures

Abbreviations: C, colon; F, fluid in peritoneal cavity; H, haustration of the colon(c); K, kerckring folds

Inflammatory Diseases

Chronic Inflammatory Intestinal Diseases

In these cases intestinal wall is thickened up to 1 cm. Sonographically stratification of bowel wall is altered, it is not disrupted in most cases. This feature helps in differentiation from carcinoma. The marginal wall which is echo-poor is most clearly thickened (Fig. 14.4). Peristalsis is slow and compressibility is reduced.

Ulcerative Diseases

There is a sonographically detectable loss of haustration, only tender echo-poor wall thickening as well as edema in the mucosa can be seen in beginning.

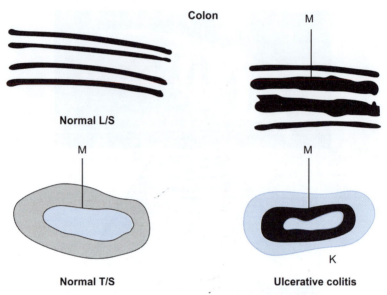

Fig. 14.4 Sonographic diagnostic criteria of ulcerative colitis (UC). Thickening of echopoor mucous membrane (M), is seen in ulcerative colitis
Abbreviations: K, cockade formation; L/S, longitudinal scan; M, mucous membrane; T/S, transverse scan

Complications requiring surgery such as paralytic and mechanical ileus and formation of fistulae and abscesses can be recognized in time by sonographic monitoring and clinical signs and laboratory tests.

Retrogression of original wall thickness to normal range (3 mm), longitudinal and transverse distention, change of layer stratification and compressibility and identification of accompanying features like fistulae, abscesses and peritonitis provide information about course of the disease.

Intussusception

The target sign is a sonographic feature of intestinal intussusception (Fig. 14.5). It appears as a double cockade formation in the lumen cross-section.

Carcinoma

By retrograde instillation of fluid sonographic assessment of the colon is significantly improved.

Irregularly limited cockade is seen in adult.

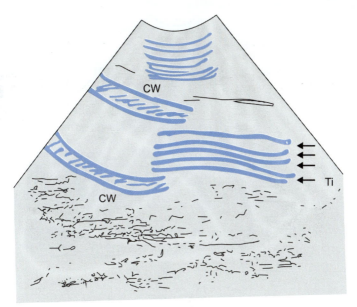

Fig. 14.5 Intussusception of terminal ileum (Ti) into the cecum. Typical sandwich phenomena of the wall layer structure in longitudinal scan on transverse scan this looks like a target sign
Abbreviation: CW, cecal wall

Target sign if visible should provide an absolute indication for surgery in adult patient.

Acute Sigmoid Diverticulitis

It is clinically describe as left sided appendicitis. The disease can be erroneously diagnosed as ureteric colic, urinary tract infection, extrauterine pregnancy, ovarian cyst or hematoma of rectus muscle.

The sigmoid colon is in close vicinity of bladder which yields an ideal contrast media for sigmoid colon. Sonographically the diverticula look like acinar appendicular structures with a hypodense sound pattern (Fig. 14.6).

Within the diverticulae particles of feces or intestinal gas can be seen.

Complications such as abscess formation, perforation, obstruction and paralysis could also be easily ascertained sonographically.

During remission, however, endoscopy is absolutely essential to exclude malignant growth.

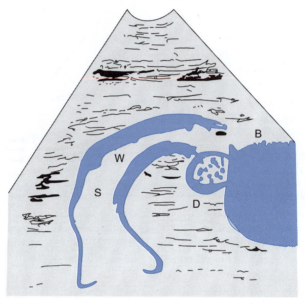

Fig. 14.6 Acute sigmoid diverticulitis (S) with long distended inflamed wall thickening (W) and typical layer stratification
Abbreviations: B, bladder; D, diverticula

Acute Appendicitis

A 5 MHz or even 7.5 MHz linear probe is used for sonographic examination of appendix.

The iliopsoas and iliac vessels which are situated medial to the appendix serve as anatomical guides.

Individually dosed compression with the scanner enables easier detection of inflamed appendix which is seen as pathological 'mini cockade' with pain evoked by compression. Occassionally intralumen fecolith is seen. Even abscess can be located. Few mildly dilated loops of small gut may be visible near iliac fossa.

Right Lower Abdominal Pain

The sonography is useful in the evaluation of right lower abdominal pain by immediate identification of an inflamed vermiform appendix and also by recognizing other diseases. These include as:
- Perforated peptic ulcer
- Torsion of ovarian cyst

- Extrauterine pregnancy
- Phlegmonous cholecystitis
- Retroperitoneal bleeding
- Crohn's disease
- Ureteric colic
- Incomplete intestinal obstruction
- Inflammation of urinary bladder.

Appendix

Acute appendicitis is one of the most frequent causes of acute abdomen in nearly all age group.

Imaging techniques such as radiographs of abdomen and barium study are of limited value. Although the normal and inflamed appendix can occassionally be seen on CT more often. The CT diagnosis of acute appendicitis is presumptive, as it depends on abscess formation or fluid collection rather than actual visualization of inflamed appendix.

Appendix is a blind ended aperistaltic tube in appendicular fossa. Normal appendix is easily compressible mobile tube. It lies anterior to common iliac artery. The normal appendix is usually not visualized.

High resolution transducer of 5–10 MHz are required to see appendix (Fig. 14.7).

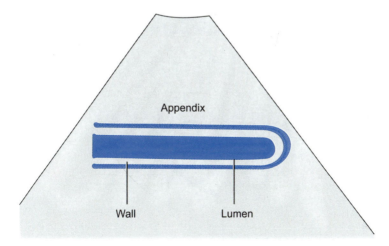

Fig. 14.7 Normal appendix—appendix is seen as well-defined thin walled tubular structure (normal up to 6 mm); lumen is anechoic

A special technique of graded compression with transducer head is applied to see the appendix. The fat and the bowels are displaced and compressed. This reduces the artifacts from bowel gas and its content. Bladder should be empty prior to the examination.

To visualize retrocecal or subhepatic appendix positions scanning should be performed both in sagittal plane through the anterior abdominal wall and in the horizontal plane from the right lateral position.

Acute Appendicitis

Appendix is seen as thick walled elongated tube with one end blind. It appears as sausage shape. When wall thickness exceeds 6 mm, it is suggestive of inflammation. Occasionally fecalith is seen in the lumen of appendix. It may be the cause of obstruction (Fig. 14.8A).

A small amount of fluid collection may be seen in appendicular fossa due to inflammation of appendix (Fig. 14.8B).

The adjacent small bowel loops may show dilatation due to local inflammation and irritation.

Local adynamic ileus may result due to inflammation.

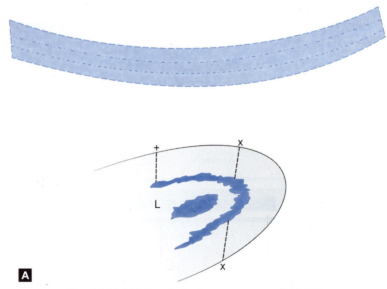

A

Fig. 14.8A Thick walled edematous appendix fluid is seen in the lumen of appendix

Abbreviations: L, lumen; x, thickened appendix; +, wall of appendix

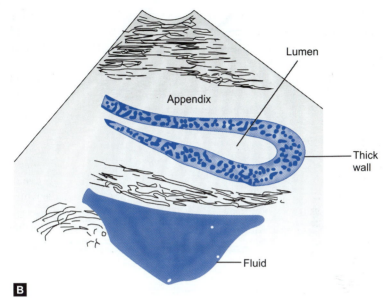

Lumen

Appendix

Thick
wall

Fluid

B

Fig. 14.8B Acute appendicitis inflamed appendix with thick edematous walls. Free fluid is seen in appendicular fossa

Appendicular Mass

Perforation of appendix leads to spill in the peritoneum, leads to peritonitis. Sometime the pus is limited due to sealing of perforation by omentum, mesentery or bowel loops.

Sonography shows noncompressible mass. It is predominantly echo poor with hetrogeneous texture.

Secondary infection may lead to an abscess formation with fluid collection and debris (Fig. 14.9).

Cecum and terminal ileum also show thickening of muscles.

Most of the abscess resolve on conservative treatment.

Differential Diagnosis of Acute Appendicitis

- Right ureteric colic
- Perforated peptic ulcer
- Right side twisted ovarian cyst
- Acute cholecystitis
- Right iliac fossa abscess
- Right side ectopic tubal pregnancy.

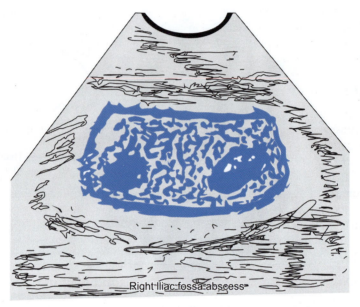

Right Iliac fossa abscess

Fig. 14.9 Abscess formation in appendiceal mass with areas of necrosis in the abscess

Limitation

Nonvisualization of appendix does not rule out appendicitis when it is aberrantly placed or retrocecal in position. In such conditions please look for indirect sign of local ileus, small fluid in appendicular fossa or an abscess formation, may lead to diagnosis.

Fluid Collections

Etiology

- Usually seromatous
- Inflammatory process
- Abscess
- Malignancy
- Trauma
  - Hematoma
  - Lymphocele
  - Urinoma.

Clinically the patient may complain pain or pain may not be present. There is bulging or bloating of skin surface due to fluid collection arising in involving subcutaneous plane, musculocutaneous plane and in intra-abdominal compartments.

Ultrasound Findings

It is variable in shapes. Fluid collection is normally anechoic. Fluid changes its position when patient changes the position with complications, the fluid becomes more complex. Sometimes septas may be seen.

Within peritoneal cavity fluid collections confirm to cavity contour.

Retroperitoneal fluid is usually lentiform or elliptically shaped, displacing kidneys.

Posterior acoustic enhancement occurs with hematoma and serous fluid but to a lesser degree with abscesses.

Abscess

Etiology

- Surgery
- Bowel perforation
- Trauma
- Pancreatitis
  Patient usually complains of pain, fever, with increase in WBC.

Ultrasound Findings

A loculated fluid collection, containing gas bubble is strongly suggestive of an abscess. This is not often seen.

More frequently one finds a fluid collection ovoid or spherical or irregular in shape, may appear thick walled; may or may not contain septation or debris.

Some abscess may simulate an echogenic solid mass or a simple cystic lesion, others show a complex appearance, partly cystic, partly solid.

The abscess is difficult to distinguish from hematoma.

Ascites

Accumulation of fluid in the peritoneal cavity is termed as ascites.

Etiology

- Transudative (due to obstruction of venous return, e.g. heart failure, cirrhosis, nephrosis)
- Exudative due to inflammation (e.g. infection, neoplasm)
- Blood, pancreatic juice, urine.

Ultrasound Findings

Free moving anechoic fluid collection is seen in abdomen. It changes its position as patient changes the position. Minimal ascites is most frequently found in hepatorenal recess (Morison's pouch) and in pelvic cul-de-sac which are the most dependent spaces of peritoneal cavity (Figs 14.10A to C).

In massive ascites liver, spleen and bowels are displaced medially and towards the center of abdomen. The bowel may appear as echogenic structures.

Loculated ascites as an isolated findings simulate mesenteric cyst, lymphocele, abscess, etc.

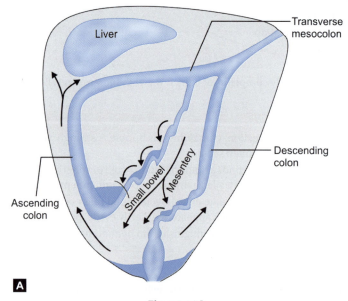

Fig. 14.10A

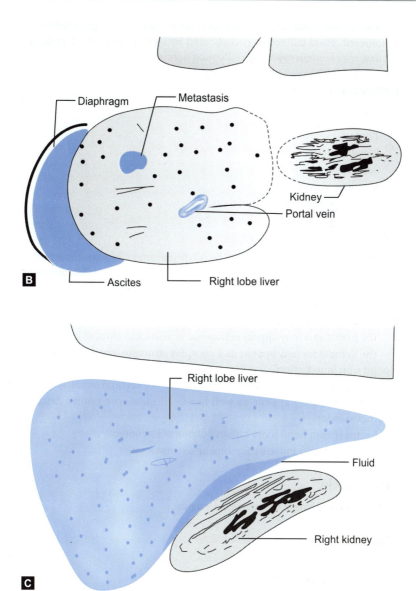

Figs 14.10B and C

Figs 14.10A to C Ascitic fluid distribution
Abbreviations: AC, ascending colon; DC, descending colon

The sonographic appearance of fluid is variable. In generally it is sonolucent. Fluid collection complicated by hemorrhage or infection or exudate may contain septation or floating debris.

Hematoma

Etiology

- Trauma
- Bleeding neoplasm
- Surgery
- Bleeding disorders.
  Patient usually complains of pain.

Ultrasound Findings

If the hematoma is small, there will be no displacement of adjacent organ. If the hematoma is large, may see distortion of adjacent organs or displacement of vena cava or aorta.

Depending upon the duration of bleeding process the change in echo pattern of hematoma is seen.

The hematoma may appear echogenic in acute and chronic hematoma.

The hematoma may appear as a complex structure when hematoma is clotted with liquefaction.

Hematoma may appear as anechoic (when serous fluid remaining).

Hematoma may appear as well localized mass or a poorly defined infiltrative lesion.

Rectus sheath hematoma causes bulging of its contour.

However, rectus muscle may appear asymptomatic.

Lymphocele

Extravasation of lymph into retroperitoneum.

Etiology

- Surgery
  - Lymphadenectomy
  - Renal transplant
- Trauma.

Ultrasound Findings

They may be small or large, asymptomatic or complicated lymphocele.

Uncomplicated lymphocele appear as echo free collection with posterior acoustic enhancement. They have smooth border. They mimic loculated ascites, mesenteric cyst or pseudopancreatic cyst.

Septation and floating debris are usually seen when they are complicated by hemorrhage or infection.

Some lymphoceles are considerable size and may cause pressure symptoms or hydronephrosis of transplant kidney (Fig. 14.11).

Urinoma

Etiology

- Surgery—renal transplant
- Trauma of kidney
- Subacute or chronic urinary obstruction resulting in perforation of collecting system

Patient may complain of decrease output of urine or palpable flank mass.

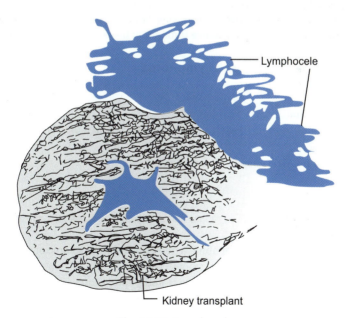

Fig. 14.11 Lymphocele

Ultrasound Findings

It is usually located in perinephric space; anechoic fluid collection with posterior acoustic enhancement.

It may have irregular border and may contain septa. May compress adjacent tissue.

Retroperitoneum

Technique

Fasting for 6–8 hours before the examination usually decreases the bowel gas that can greatly interfere with visualization of retroperitoneum. In most adults 3.5 MHz transducer will provide adequate penetration for evaluation of retroperitoneum. The evaluation of retroperitoneum should be done in both transverse and longitudinal planes, in supine and lateral decubitus positions. Initial sonographic evaluation of retroperitoneum, is performed with subject in a supine position. The great vessels are identified in midline and the para-aortic and paracaval region are examined from the level of diaphragm to, and including the iliac vessels.

Generally the aorta enters the abdominal cavity for posterior but becomes progressively more anterior as it travels caudally. The inferior vena cava maintain a more horizontal course throughout the peritoneum.

Lymphadenopathy and Lymphoma

Etiology

- Lymphoma
- Metastatic tumors (testicle, renal cells, uterus, ovary, etc.)
- Infection
- AIDS and AIDS-related diseases.

Ultrasound Findings

Lymph nodes more than 1 cm can be visualized in para-aortic, mesenteric and celiac nodes.

The lymph nodes appear homogeneous, mainly hypoechoic or anechoic with low level echogenicity and smooth borders.

There is no correlation between node appearance and lymphoma histology. No posterior acoustic enhancement is seen (Fig. 14.12A).

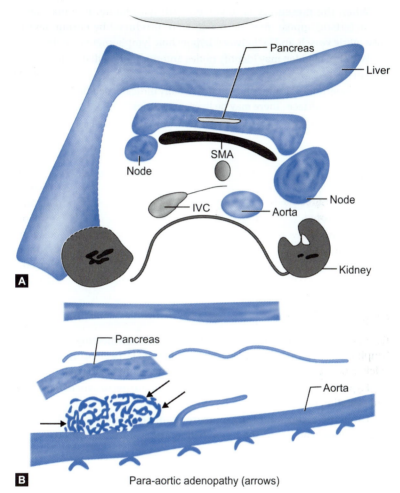

Para-aortic adenopathy (arrows)

Figs 14.12A and B Lymphadenopathy and lymphoma
Abbreviations: IVC, inferior vena cava; SMA, superior mesenteric artery

As nodes enlarge they may become irregular in shape and may displace surrounding anatomy. Lymph nodes may present as multiple, septate lobulated lymph nodes (more than 1–2 cm sizes).

Nodes may appear as bulky conglomerate mass of enlarged lymph nodes.

Para-aortic lymph nodes frequently obscure the echogenic anterior aortic border producing a 'sonographic silhouette' which helps distinguish para-aortic disease from mesenteric nodes (Fig. 14.12B).

When the mesentery is involved with lymphoma, one may see a characteristic appearance 'sandwich sign' produced by entrapment of mesenteric vessels and fat between hypoechoic lymphomatous nodes.

With full bladder, may identify nodes anterior and medial to iliac vessel margins.

Retroperitoneal tumor plus ascites usually indicates seeding or invasion of peritoneal surface. There may be liver metastases.

Masses

Etiology

Primary tumors are:
- Leiomyosarcoma
- Liposarcoma
- Fibrosarcoma
- Neuroblastoma
- Rhabdomyosarcoma
- Teratoma.

Ultrasound Findings

Retroperitoneal malignancies are ill defined and more heterogeneous than lymphomas. Increase echogenicity may be related to fat content (liposarcoma) calcification, vascularity (Hemangiopericytoma) or hemorrhage.

Hypoechogenicity or cystic portion may be due to necrosis or hemorrhage and septation may be seen.

Dramatic distortion of organ anatomy displacement or. indentation of great vessels are seen. The lesion will not be distorted when pressure is applied by transducer.

Retroperitoneal Fibrosis

Etiology

- Unknown
- May be idiopathic, related to infiltrating neoplasm or acute immune disease.

Ultrasound Findings

Discrete, hypoechoic mass of smooth contoured tissue lying anterior and lateral to great vessels.

15

Ultrasonography of the Scrotum

Ultrasound Appearances of Scrotum

Normal Scrotum (Transverse section)

The testicular parenchymal echo pattern is even and similar to that of thyroid, i.e. finely granular echogenicity. Median raphe (central) is an area of high attenuation. The ductus deferens is visualized along the posterior medial aspect of each testis as a relatively circular echo-free area (Fig. 15.1).

Longitudinal scan of testes are usually best performed with a contact scanner after palpable epididymis has been aligned directly posterior to the glandular element of the testes. The superficial scrotal area can be appreciated and the potential space created by tunica vaginalis can often be seen as an echogenic line. The fine homogeneous texture of glandular element of testes is even more evident (Fig. 15.2).

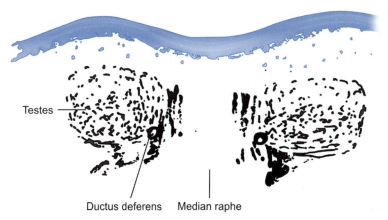

Testes

Ductus deferens   Median raphe

Fig. 15.1 Normal scrotum (Transverse section)

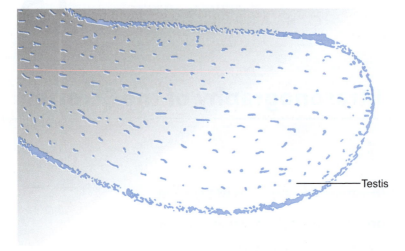

Fig. 15.2 Testis (Longitudinal section)

The echogenic tubular structure in mid portion of testicular parenchymal echoes are due to tunica vaginalis and mediastinum testis which contain testicular vessels running through the mid portion of gland (Fig. 15.3). The normal epididymis is usually 7–8 mm thick and lies posterolateral to testes. Its echogenicity is similar to that of testes although the parenchymal texture is somewhat coarses. The head (globus major) lies adjacent to superior pole of testes and constitutes the joining of 10–15 efferent ducts from testes into a single duct. The body and tail of epididymis course lateral and progressively inferior to the testes, where the tail of epididymis is invested with a muscular coat and ascends medially as the ductus deferens.

Testicular Masses

Separation of intratesticular and extratesticular pathology is the most valuable diagnostic clue provided by scrotal sonography.

Malignant

Seminomas: These tumors are usually homogeneously hypoechoic with a paucity of necrosis or hemorrhage (Figs 15.4 and 15.5).

Occasionally the tumor involves nearly the entire gland (Fig. 15.6).

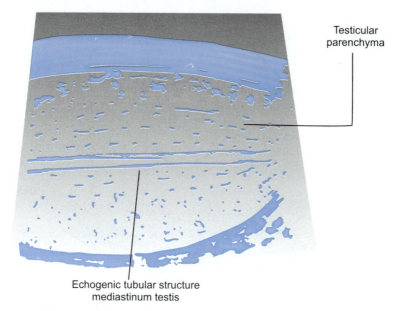

Testicular
parenchyma

Echogenic tubular structure
mediastinum testis

Fig. 15.3 Midportion of testicular gland (Longitudinal section)

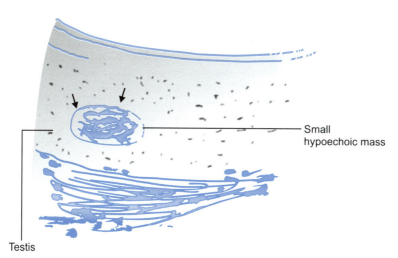

Small
hypoechoic mass

Testis

Fig. 15.4 Seminoma—testes (Longitudinal section)

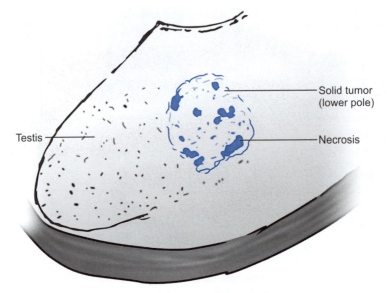

Fig. 15.5 Necrosis in tumor

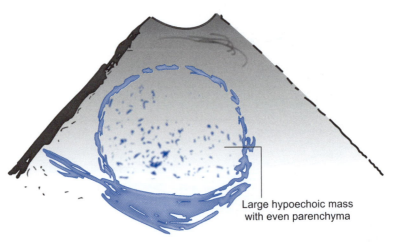

Fig. 15.6 Large seminoma—testes (Transverse section)

Whenever a lesion involves the entire gland and has a fairly even parenchymal pattern. It can easily be missed. Please compare echo pattern of testes from normal testes.

Embryonal cell carcinoma: Less well-circumscribed hypoechoic masses that are more in-homogeneous than seminomas. These often contains areas of hemorrhagic necrosis or cystic changes.

Testicular metastases: These are multiple bilateral lesions which are indistinguishable in appearance from primary testicular tumor. They arise from genitourinary tract, lung and pancreas.

Lymphoma or leukemia: They may be focal hypoechoic lesions or diffuse hypoechoic enlargement of the testes (Fig. 15.7).

Benign

Testicular abscess: It is secondary to epididymo-orchitis often occurring in diabetic patient. Sonographically abscess are hypoechoic or complex masses. They may rupture into tunica vaginalis and lead to pyocele formation.

Testicular Infarct: They can result from trauma, infection, torsion.

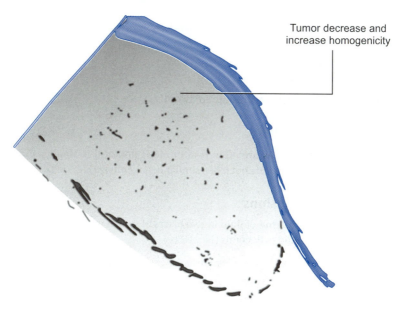

Tumor decrease and increase homogenicity

Fig. 15.7 Testicular tumor (Lymphoma-leukemia) (Longitudinal section)

These infarcts may present as focal hypoechoic masses or as diffusely hypoechoic small testes.

Occasionally, echogenic area may be seen in infarct. This could be due to focal fibrosis.

Acute Scrotum

Torsion of Testes

It results from torsion of spermatic cord. The sonographically the typical features of involvement of entire scrotum, a reactive hydrocele and abnormal acoustic texture to the glandular element of testes.

Trauma of Testes

Hemorrhagic hydrocele demonstrate the complex mass surrounding the glandular element of testes. The two testes appear unequal in size and acoustic texture.

Acute Epididymis

Sonographic changes are enlarged hypoechoic epididymis associated with otherwise normal testes.

In 20% of cases in epididymis focal hypoechoic area of testicular orchitis or testicular enlargement (Fig. 15.8).

Chronic Epididymis

It may result in enlarged echogenic epididymis.

Undescended Testes

The undescended testes are often oval or elongated and is smaller than normally positioned glands but it has similar echogenicity (Fig. 15.9).

Extratesticular Lesions

Hydrocele: Accumulation of fluid in two layers of tunica vaginalis. They are usually anechoic fluid collections (Fig. 15.10).

Hematocele: It often contains septation and loculation with dependent debris.

Varicocele: They are dilated veins of pampiniform plexus and usually lie posterolateral to testes. They are hypoechoic tubular lucencies (Fig. 15.11).

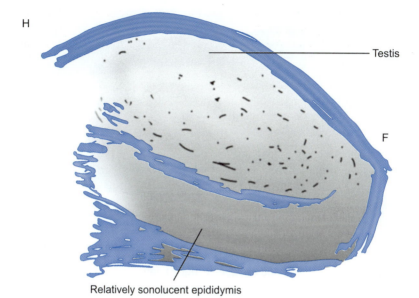

Fig. 15.8 Acute epididymitis (Longitudinal section)
Abbreviations: H, head; F, foot

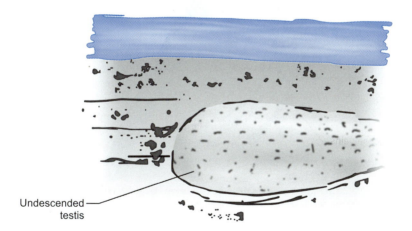

Fig. 15.9 Undescended testis—right inguinal region (Longitudinal section)

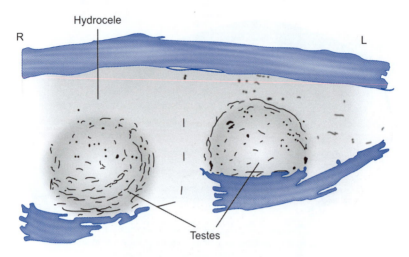

Fig. 15.10 Hydrocele (Longitudinal section)
Abbreviations: R, right; L, left

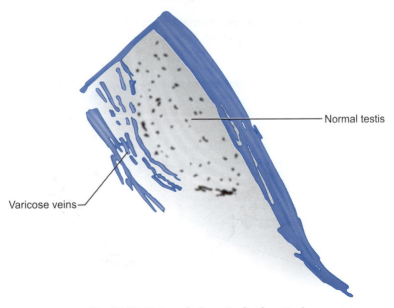

Fig. 15.11 Varicocele (Longitudinal section)

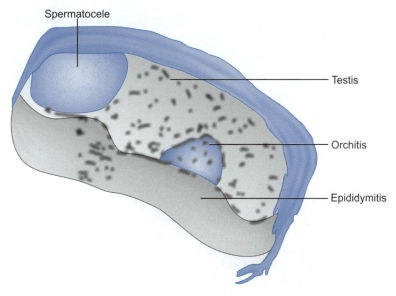

Fig. 15.12 Spermatocele, epididymitis or orchitis (Longitudinal section)

Spermatocele: They are most common in the region of globus major. They are cyst contain fluid with spermatozoa. The range in size of few mm to cm (Fig. 15.12).

CHAPTER 16

Ultrasonography of the Thyroid

Thyroid Gland

The normal thyroid gland is a highly vascular organ consisting of two larger lateral lobes and a connecting isthmus of variable size. It is approximately 5 cm long, 3 cm wide, and weights 20–30 g. The right lobe is usually slightly larger than the left. Rarely, an entire lobe may be absent as a result of agenesis. When this occurs, absence of the left lobe is most common. In at least 15% of the population, a pyramidal lobe is present extending from the isthmus or the medical aspect of one of the upper poles (Fig. 16.1).

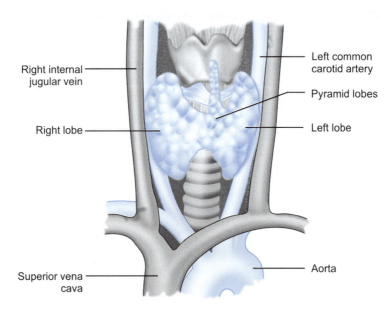

Fig. 16.1 Thyroid gland: anterior view

The thyroid is situated in the neck, immediately anterior to the trachea and inferior to the thyroid cartilage of the larynx. In cases where partial agenesis occurs, remnants of normally located or ectopic thyroid tissue is found. Of the ectopic locations, approximately half are localized at the base of the tongue (lingual, intralingual, or sublingual thyroid), and the remainder are found between the tongue and sternum.

The thyroid is supplied with blood from the right and left superior and right and left inferior thyroid arteries, which are branches of the external carotid arteries. Its blood supply is drained into the internal jugular veins by the superior and middle thyroid veins, and into the innominate veins by the inferior thyroid veins.

Thyroid tissue is composed of basic functioning units called follicles, each follicle consists of an acinar wall of closely packed cuboidal epithelial cells surrounding a central lumen. The follicles rest directly on interfollicular connective tissue containing blood and lymph capillaries. Dispersed within the follicles are the parafollicular cells, sometimes referred to as C cells.

Pathology

Thyroid abnormalities may result from the gland producing either, excess or a diminished output of thyroid hormone. Hypersecretion results in hyperthyroidism, and hyposecretion, hypothyroidism. Other categories of thyroid disease include those conditions that do not produce a recognizable effect on hormone production (e.g. carcinoma) and conditions simulating true inflammation, such as thyroiditis.

An enlargement of the thyroid, known as goiter, is present in many different types of thyroid disease. Enlargement may be generalized or focal. Generalized enlargements, however, are not always symmetrical. The right lobe tends to enlarge more than the left. True focal enlargement usually indicate neoplastic transformation, either malignant or benign.

Thyroid diseases of all categories are common in area of iodine deficiency and rare in regions of high iodine intake.

Hyperthyroidism

Hyperthyroidism, clinically known as thyrotoxicosis, refers to the state of heightened metabolic activity caused by an excess of thyroid hormone. It is most commonly the result of a condition known as Graves' disease, and is seen most often in females and may be related to emotional trauma. Graves' disease can also be caused by excessive thyroid hormone production, and single toxic nodule, a toxic multinodular goiter, occasionally functioning thyroid carcinomas, or medication. Hypertrophy and hyperplasia of the thyroid follicles are the principal findings, thus the patient usually presents with a goiter. The patient may exhibit some or all of the clinical manifestations of hyperthyroids, which may include an elevated metabolic rate, exophthalmos, nervousness and irritability, menstrual changes, elevated body temperature, increased sensitivity to heat with nearly continuous perspiration, diarrhea, weight loss with increased appetite, palpitations, muscle weakness, and a fine tremor 'in the hands.'

Hypothyroidism

Hypothyroidism refers to the hypometabolic state characterized by the progressive slowing of all bodily functions as a result of inadequate circulating levels of thyroid hormone.

Hypothyroidism may be primary due to failure of the thyroid, or secondary due to diseases of the hypothalamus of pituitary.

In adults who acquire hypothyroidism usually do so as a result of Hashimoto's thyroiditis. In the adult, signs and symptoms of thyroid deficiency are nonspecific, and their onset may be subtle. They include a slowing of intellectual and motor performance, cold intolerance, nervousness and menorrhagia. More specific changes, when present include a bloated appearance, with thickened; dry cold, edematous skin; weight gain; and an enlarged heart.

Endemic Goiter

Endemic goiter, then may be defined as any enlargement of the thyroid gland that does not result from an inflammatory or neoplastic process and is not initially associated with thyrotoxicosis or acquired hypothyroidism. Other terms for this enlargement are simple goiter and nontoxic goiter.

Iodine deprivation is thought to cause a reduction in thyroid hormone production, which is sensed by the pituitary, which then achieves a level of feedback by secreting augmented quantities of thyroid-stimulating hormone (TSH). This results in an increased iodine uptake by the thyroid as the gland strives to gain the necessary 60–100 mg of iodine needed daily for hormonogenesis. The follicles become hyperplastic, and a diffuse, symmetrical enlargement of the gland results. Eventually, the thyroid may become multinodular.

The frequency of simple goiter peaks during puberty, and girls are affected more often than boys.

Multinodular Goiter

Multinodular goiter refers to a thyroid enlargement associated with more than one nodule. These goiters are generally the largest type encountered, weighing up to 1000 g, with nodules ranging in size from 0.5 cm to several centimeters in diameter. The enlargement is frequently asymmetrical and expansion may occur downward behind the sternum to produce an intrathoracic or retrosternal goiter.

Although the etiology of multinodular goiter is not known with certainty, one cause may be a mild deficiency in thyroid hormone production with consequent long-standing stimulation of the thyroid by TSH. It is frequently the result of a long-standing simple goiter. Because there is a high familial incidence, the cause may be an inherited partial defect in hormone synthesis.

Neoplasms

Thyroid neoplasms are divided into two groups; adenomas, and malignant tumors. The adenomas vary greatly in size and histologic characteristics and are classified into three major types; follicular, papillary, and Hurthle cells. The four principal varieties of thyroid carcinoma are papillary, follicular, anaplastic and medullary.

Thyroid Adenomas

These new growths of thyroid tissue have a homogeneous histologic pattern, are encapsulated, and usually compress contiguous tissue. They may be present as single mass in otherwise normal glands or as multiple discrete structures. They may also be included as part of a multinodular goiter.

Of the three major benign thyroid neoplasms, follicular adenomas are the most common. They are the most highly differentiated and most likely to mimic normal thyroid tissue. They usually present as solitary nodules that have been growing slowly over a period of many years. Adenomas may concentrate radioactive iodine to varying degrees, and on nuclear medicine scans they may appear 'warm', or 'hot'. If they undergo hemorrhagic necrosis, resulting in loss of function, they become 'cold'. At this stage, the adenoma has a cystic component filled with a gelatinous material.

Thyroid Carcinomas

Thyroid carcinomas are of two varieties; those arising in the follicular epithelium, and those arising in the parafollicular, or C cells. Carcinomas of the follicular epithelium are of three histologic types, which differ in their clinical course. Nearly 80% are papillary tumors; these usually grow slowly and typically spread to the regional lymph nodes, where they remain for many years. Eventually, metastasis can occur in the strap muscles, larynx, and lungs. The lesions of papillary carcinoma are usually solitary, but may also be multifocal, ranging from microscopic foci to areas up to 10 cm in diameter.

Follicular and anaplastic carcinomas account for the remainder of follicular epithelium carcinomas. Most commonly, follicular carcinomas present as a slowly enlarging, irregular lump, often in an already nodular gland. Anaplastic carcinomas are usually seen as bulky masses which have invaded beyond the thyroid capsule.

Medullary carcinomas tend to metastasis locally to the neck, and to the lungs and soft tissue.

Thyroiditis

The term thyroiditis encompasses several disorders of differing etiology, the two most common being subacute thyroiditis and Hashimoto's disease.

Subacute thyroiditis, also known as granulomatosis, or giant cell thyroiditis, is an inflammatory condition thought to be of viral origin, usually causing exquisite tenderness and enlargement over the thyroid. The pain may radiate to the head, arms, and chest. It may be unilateral at the onset, but it usually migrates to involve the entire gland. The disease tends to remit spontaneously, and over a 1–12 months period, subsides completely.

Ultrasound

Patients who have had 'warm' or 'cold' areas demonstrated on their nuclear medicine scan then, should have an ultrasonic thyroid evaluation. Using the classical criteria established for cyst recognition, the scan will determine if the nodule in question is cystic or solid.

Before his/her ultrasonic scan, the patient's thyroid is palpated to define specific areas of interest. He is then typically placed in the supine position with the neck hyperextended. Either a water-path, or a conducting gel of low viscosity is used as a coupling agent. Sagittal and transverse scans of the entire gland are then obtained.

The transducer should have a frequency of at least 5 MHz, and should be focussed close to the skin's surface because of the thyroid's superficiality. Scanning technique must be meticulous.

The internal structure of the normal thyroid is seen as a fine, homogenous echopattern of a medium gray tone. The common carotid arteries are seen immediately posterior and lateral to the thyroid's right and left lobes. Lateral to these are the jugular veins (Figs 16.2 and 16.3).

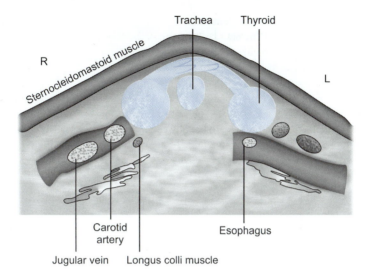

Fig. 16.2 Normal thyroid (Transverse section)
Abbreviations: R, right; L, left

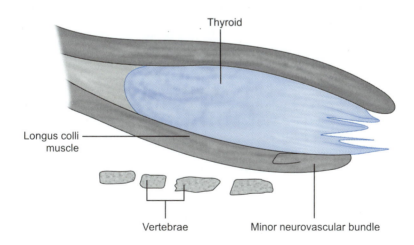

Fig. 16.3 Normal thyroid (Longitudinal section)

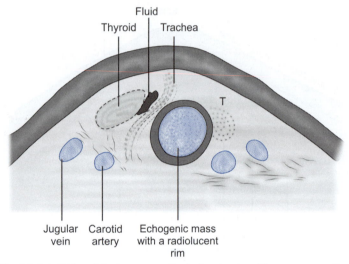

Fig. 16.4 Left thyroid adenoma—displacing trachea (Transverse section)
Abbreviation: T, trachea

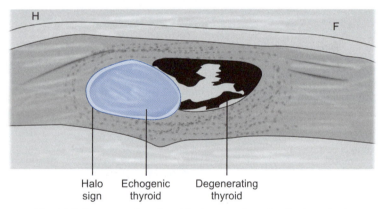

Fig. 16.5 Degenerating thyroid adenoma (Longitudinal section)
Abbreviations: F, foot side; H, head side

Thyroid adenomas present as well-circumscribed lesions of varying diameter. The internal echopattern is homogenous and fine with the echogenecity varying from a more to a less echogenic pattern than that of normal thyroid tissue. If the lesion has undergone degeneration, small, irregular, anechoic areas representing hemorrhagic or cystic change will be seen. Frequently a well-defined rim or 'halo' is seen surrounding the periphery of the nodule (Figs 16.4 and 16.5).

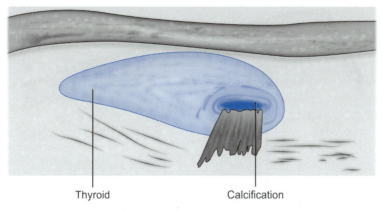

Thyroid   Calcification

Fig. 16.6 Calcified thyroid adenoma (Longitudinal section)

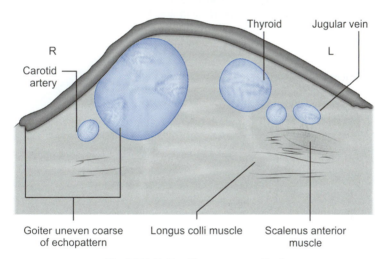

Thyroid   Jugular vein

R   L

Carotid
artery

Goiter uneven coarse   Longus colli muscle   Scalenus anterior
   of echopattern   muscle

Fig. 16.7 Goiter (Transverse section)
Abbreviations: R, right; L, left

Goiters can appear as either discrete masses, or diffuse lesions involving an entire lobe or gland. As with adenomas, a peripheral halo and fluid filled areas representing internal cystic degeneration are sometimes seen. The lesions echogenicity, however is most often equivalent to that of normal thyroid parenchyma. When areas of calcification are present, they will stand out as prominent, reflective echoes with sharply demarcated acoustic shadows deep to the areas of calcification (Figs 16.6 and 16.7).

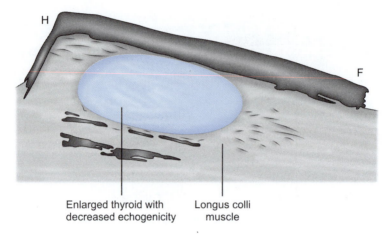

Enlarged thyroid with   Longus colli
decreased echogenicity   muscle

Fig. 16.8 Thyroiditis (Longitudinal section)
Abbreviations: H, head side; F, foot side

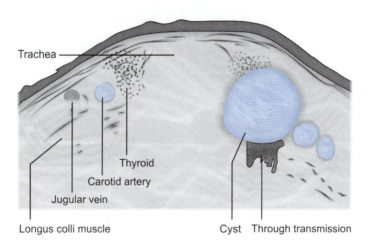

Trachea

Thyroid

Carotid artery

Jugular vein

Longus colli muscle   Cyst   Through transmission

Fig. 16.9A Thyroid cyst (Transverse section)

Common sonographic features of thyroiditis, include an enlarged gland with a generalized decrease in echogenicity (Fig. 16.8).

If a cyst is demonstrated, the patient can be followed with repeat ultrasound examination to monitor its size or the cyst can be aspirated under ultrasonic guidance and the fluid examined for malignant cells (Figs 16.9A and 16.9B). When a solid lesion is found by ultrasound, surgery or percutaneous

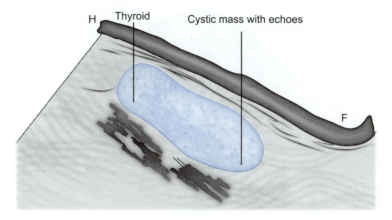

Fig. 16.9B Hemorrhagic cyst (Longitudinal section)
Abbreviations: H, head side; F, foot side

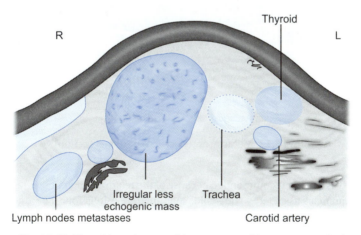

Fig. 16.10 Thyroid carcinoma with metastases (Transverse section)
Abbreviations: R, right; L, left

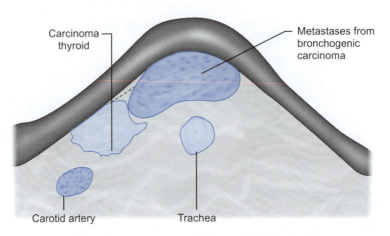

Fig. 16.11 Thyroid carcinoma (Transverse section)

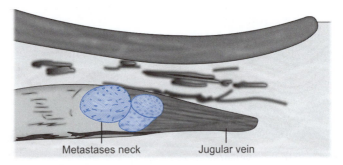

Fig. 16.12 Metastases—neck (Longitudinal section)

biopsy is usually recommended because of the relatively high percentage of malignancies associated with 'cold', solid thyroid lesions found on nuclear medicine scans (Figs 16.10 to 16.12).

17

Breast

Anatomy

The breast is composed of 15–20 lobes. Each opens individually via lactiferous duct on to the surface of nipple. These ducts can be visualized in the lactating breast.

The deep pectoral fascia is seen on the deep aspect of breast overlying the pectoralis major muscle.

The lobes are divided by fibrous partitions which constitute the Cooper's ligaments. These fibrous strands pass from deep pectoral fascia and through the breast to be inserted into skin. With increasing age more fat is seen infiltrating the breast and less glandular tissue (Figs 17.1 and 17.2).

The postmenopausal fatty breast appears rather featureless on ultrasound.

Lactating Breast

There is hypertrophy of glandular tissue and the lactiferous ducts become distended with milk.

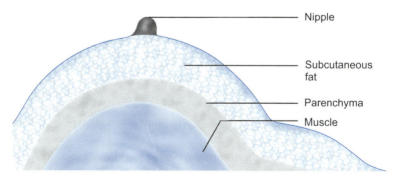

Fig. 17.1 Normal anatomy—breast

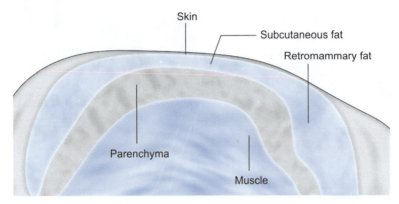

Fig. 17.2 Breast (Transverse section)

Ultrasound shows pectoralis major muscle on the deep surface of breast covered by deep pectoral fascia. The breast tissue is uniform apart except from tubular disruptions due to dilated lactiferous duct.

Hypertrophy

Ultrasound scan demonstrates normal rather echogenic glandular tissue in the region of palpable mass.

The hypertrophy could be due to secretion of excessive estrogen which can lead to increased fibroglandular tissue formations.

Fibrocystic Disease

On palpation, the breast feels lumpy with or without dominant mass.

Ultrasound examination shows only very dense tissue with or without the evidence of cyst. These dense areas presumably are of fibrous mastopathy-benign in origin.

Sometimes small cystic areas may present a honeycomb appearance of microcystic disease (Fig. 17.3).

Nonpalpable Mass

Large cysts of breast may be present but may not be palpable. They are well demonstrated by ultrasound.

Ultrasound examination may reveal cystic area in the breast. In some cases, the fluid could be moved by palpation freely. Flaccidity of cyst is responsible for the lack of palpability of mass (Fig. 17.4).

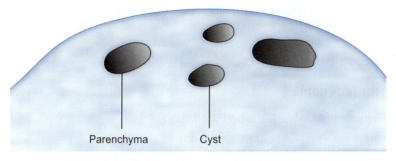

Fig. 17.3 Multiple cysts (sagittal whole breast section)

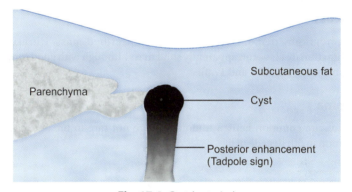

Fig. 17.4 Cyst (anterior)

Aspiration

On palpation, the breast a freely mobile mass is present. Xeroradiography, however, may not show the mass. Ultrasound examination demonstrates a cystic mass. Ultrasound prior to attempted aspiration is valuable in diagnosing the presence of cystic rather than a solid mass. Enormous relief is often achieved by the simple procedure of aspiration which is both diagnostic and therapeutic.

Calcified Cysts

Ill-defined lumps presented in the breast. Mammography can show multiple rings of calcification consistent with calcified cysts or fat necrosis.

Ultrasound scan demonstrates the cystic areas as well as with marked shadowing from their wall.

Benign Tumors

Fibroadenoma

Firm, Freely Mobile Mass on Palpitation

Ultrasound examination reveals well-defined oval or round apparently echogenic mass. There is a good through transmission. No evidence of spread into the surrounding tissue. It may cause compression to the surrounding tissue. It is avascular on Doppler study (Figs 17.5 and 17.6).

Abscess

Mammography demonstrates a well circumscribed mass. Ultrasound examination discloses an apparently solid mass although with good through transmission (Figs 17.7 and 17.8).

Lipoma

Lipoma are common benign tumors and are not rare in breast. They are common in 5th decade of life.

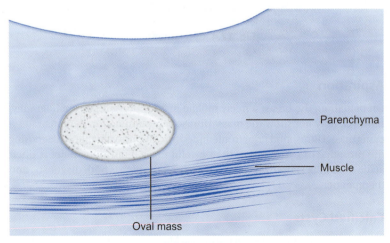

Parenchyma

Muscle

Oval mass

Fig. 17.5 Fibroadenoma (Longitudinal section)

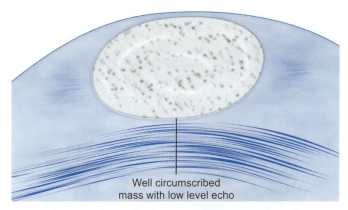

Fig. 17.6 Large fibroadenoma (in pregnant breast)

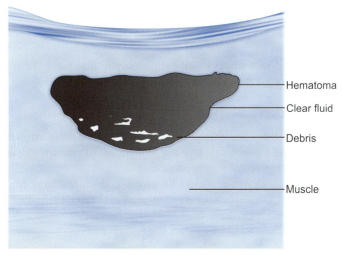

Fig. 17.7 Hematoma (Longitudinal section)

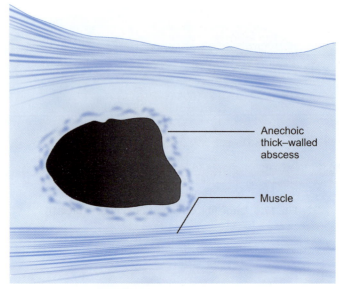

Fig. 17.8 Abscess (Longitudinal section)

Ultrasound demonstrates a well-defined, hypoechoic mass. The fibrous stroma can be traced through the mass.

Inspissated Cyst

Mammography shows dense tissue without any dominant mass. Inspissation of the contents of a galactocele give rise to material with the consistency of toothpaste with high acoustic impedance.

Ultrasound scan demonstrates an acoustic shadow arising from an echogenic mass. This shadowing is reminiscent of that seen in some breast cancer.

Carcinoma

The malignant tumors are mostly solid, irregular in outline. There may be infiltration of adjacent soft tissue.

Xeromammography shows poorly defined density, retraction of nipple and thickening of skin in mass lying anteriorly. If the mass is invading posteriorly then one can see disruption of the retromammary fat line and a probable invasion of pectoral muscle or tentacles invading the adjacent breast.

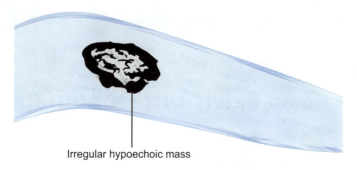

Irregular hypoechoic mass

Fig. 17.9 Breast malignancy (ductal carcinoma) (Longitudinal section)

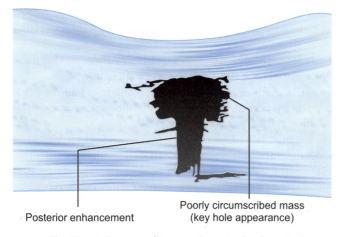

Posterior enhancement

Poorly circumscribed mass (key hole appearance)

Fig. 17.10 Breast malignancy (Longitudinal section)

Ultrasound demonstrates, almost invariably hypoechoic although varying degree of echogenicity may be seen in scirrhous carcinoma. Mass is mainly irregular and ill-defined. Increased attenuation with distal shadowing is seen (Figs 17.9 and 17.10).

Lymphoma

Ultrasound examination reveals solid, irregular, hypoechoic masses.

Pelvic Ultrasonography

Female Pelvis: Technique

Full urinary bladder is essential for adequate pelvic sonogram. A full bladder provides an acoustic window, displaces the uterus to less anteverted position, allowing easier sonographic visualization, displace air fluid bowel out of true pelvis.

Over-distended bladder not only causes patient discomfort but it also may distort the uterine shape and displace masses out of true pelvis.

Most pelvic scanning can be performed medium or long focus 3.5 MHz transducer. The overall gain should be set so that there are no echoes in bladder and medium amplitude echoes in the uterus.

First a longitudinal midline scan is performed to check bladder distention. The bladder should be sufficiently distended to allow adequate visualization of uterine fundus, through the bladder. If the bladder distention is satisfactory the longitudinal scans are obtained throughout the entire pelvis. When studying the uterus, it is important to keep the transducer angled perpendicular to the long axis of uterus to allow visualization of the specular echo from the endometrial cavity.

Transverse sections from the symphysis pubis in cephaloid-directions are performed at 1 cm interval.

The ovaries are identified in transverse/oblique scans, 0.5 cm interval images through them should be obtained. Uterus is not always located in midline and this can be accentuated in distention. Oblique longitudinal scans should than be performed along the long axis of uterus. Straight longitudinal scan with scan angled laterally are sometimes helpful in identifying the ovaries in longitudinal plane.

Bowel in pelvis can be identified by peristalsis. Sometimes, it is difficult to separate bowel from other pelvic structures or pelvic masses. In these cases, water enema can be performed.

Uterus

Roughly the shape of a small pear, the uterus is a hollow, muscular pouch suspended by the broad ligaments, located between the bladder and the rectum, in the pelvis, normally weighing only 2 oz. The uterus is capable of playing a key role in the most staggering accomplishment of our universe: the protection and nourishment of a barely visible cluster of cells which eventually multiply more than a trillion times to become a human being.

The uterus is divided into three main parts: body or corpus (the main portion); base or fundus (lying above the opening of the oviducts or fallopian tubes) which forms the upper, dome-shaped portion; and the cervix, which projects into the vagina.

The uterus consists of three layers: (1) outer (called the serous or perimetrium); (2) middle (muscular layer called the myometrium and (3) inner (mucous layer) called the endometrium.

Each month dazzling displays of chemistry take place to signal the construction of intricate networks of new blood vessels, tissue and glands. Prompted by estrogen hormones secreted by the ovaries, the blood-red, velvety smooth inner lining (endometrium) thickens, preparing the essential nourishment for possible new life. At midcycle the ovaries begin producing the hormone progesterone which performs several helpful functions: preparation of the lining of the uterus for implantation and secretion (by the glands already stimulated by estrogen) of nutritional substances to sustain the fertilized egg during its early growth stages. The progesterone also acts to relax the muscles of the uterus to prevent expulsion of the fertilized egg. Normally uterine muscles contract regularly.

There are three openings to the uterus. Two fallopian tubes feed into the upper portion of the uterus. These tubes are about 10 cm long but only 0.625 cm (1/4″) wide. They lie in the broad ligaments and emerge from the uterus at the junction of the body and fundus. They curve horizontally and backward to reach the ovaries, which they overlap. It is the function of the tube to provide the passage way and muscular movement necessary to propel the fertilized egg into the uterus (Fig. 18.1).

Each of the tubes is divided into four parts:
1. *Interstitial:* Short portion that passes through uterine wall
2. *Isthmus:* Medial portion
3. *Ampulla:* Widest, longest and thinnest walled (therefore dilatable)
4. *Infundibulum:* Trumpet-shaped, expanded outer portion whose extreme surface is broken up into numerous finger-like processes called fimbriae.

The third opening to the uterus is a straw-sized tunnel through the cervix, or neck of the uterus. This entrance serves as the entrance for sperm and

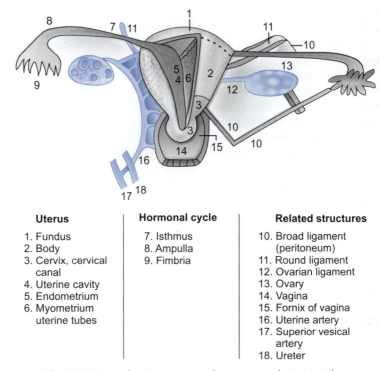

Uterus	Hormonal cycle	Related structures
1. Fundus	7. Isthmus	10. Broad ligament
2. Body	8. Ampulla	(peritoneum)
3. Cervix, cervical	9. Fimbria	11. Round ligament
canal		12. Ovarian ligament
4. Uterine cavity		13. Ovary
5. Endometrium		14. Vagina
6. Myometrium		15. Fornix of vagina
uterine tubes		16. Uterine artery
		17. Superior vesical
		artery
		18. Ureter

Fig. 18.1 Reproductive system—the uterus and uterine tubes

the exit for the fetus. Simultaneously with ovulation, the cervix produces an increased amount of fluid from its mucous glands to provide a stream through which the sperm can swim towards the egg.

If no fertilized egg is received all of the new tissues, glands and blood vessels are shed or cast off in the process called menstruation. Not infrequently, this event is accompanied by cramping pains called *dysmenorrhea*. If the uterine lining does not develop or slough off properly each month, excessive or irregular bleeding results. Correction of this condition is the widely used surgical technique-dilatation and curettage (D and C) in which the cervix is dilated by instruments to scrap away the condition which usually disappears.

Uterine cancer (of the lining or the cervix) ranks only second to breast cancer as the most common site of female cancer. It is usually readily detectable and if treated early enough has over 90% cure rate. Abnormal bleeding after age 40 is the most frequent symptom of endometrial cancer and while it may be related to other things, it should be reported to the physician immediately. The pap test has proven an invaluable diagnostic aid in detection of cervical cancer and should be repeated yearly. It should be repeated every six months in females taking birth control pills.

Normal Anatomy

Uterus (Figs 18.2 and 18.3)

Position Uterus is located in the midline between bladder and rectum.

Size Prepubertal uterus—(Longitudinal)—2.0–3.5 cm long, 0.5–1.0 cm wide.

Postpubertal uterus—4–7 cm long, 4.0 cm wide. Multiparity increases the normal size 1.2 cm in all directions.

Postmenopausal—3.5–6.5 cm long, 1.2–1.8 cm wide.

Shape Prepubertal uterus

The cervix makes up to 2/3–5/6 of total uterine length

Postpubertal uterus

Fundus is larger and longer than cervix.

Contour Uterus is normally smooth in contour and distinctly outlined.

Texture Uterus shows homogenous low to moderate echogenicity.

Central Uterine Cavity Echo

Within the uterus, there is centrally located linear echo of moderate to high amplitude. The echo may not show in retroverted uteri, in which uterine cavity is not perpendicular to sound beam (Fig. 18.4).

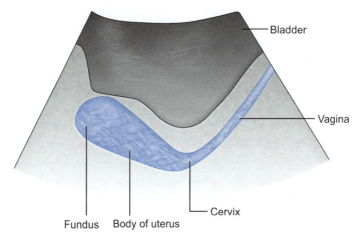

Fig. 18.2 Normal anatomy (Longitudinal section)

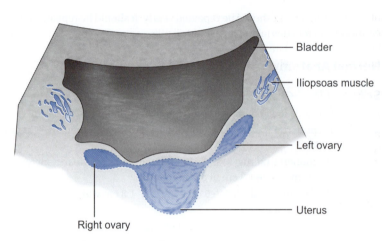

Fig. 18.3 Normal anatomy (Transverse section)

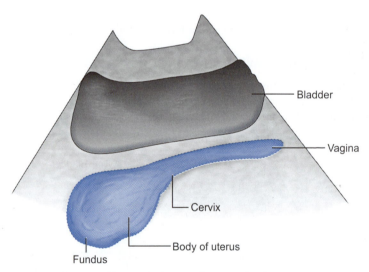

Fig. 18.4 Retroverted uterus (Longitudinal section)

Often 2–3 mm zone of low amplitude echoes, surrounds the central cavity echo. It is believed to represent the endometrium.

Identifying the central uterine cavity echo establishes conclusively which structure represents the uterus and which structure represents the extrauterine masses. A pelvic mass that touches the central uterine cavity echo must be uterine in origin. The presence of normal central uterine cavity echo may also help show that the uterus is nongravid and empty. The central cavity echo may be increased in thickness or echogenicity with various endometrial alterations. Endometrial hyperplasia and polyps typically produce this ultrasound pattern.

Sonographic Morphology of the Normal Menstrual Cycle

Ultrasound examination was performed at three sequential points in the menstrual cycle, ovulation, midluteal phase, and menses. The first sonogram was obtained within 48 hours of ovulation, the second 7–10 days later during the midluteal phase, and the third during the subsequent menses.

Ovaries: The ovaries showed the most variation during the three sequential examinations. Ovarian cysts were readily identified throughout the cycle. The cysts were of two different sizes. Smaller cysts measuring 0.6–1.5 cm in diameter (mean 1.0 cm). Larger cysts ranging from 1.6–2.4 cm in diameter (mean 2.2 cm) were identified in the midluteal phase.

Uterus: In contrast to the complex ovarian changes, uterine ultrasonic morphology remains relatively constant except for a characteristic hypoechoic transformation during the midluteal stage. Midluteal studies disclose a "bull's-eye" uterine configuration of the uterus on the transverse images, characterized by an outer echo genic area (myometrium) with a more hypoechoic inner region (endometrium) and a high-amplitude central-echo complex (mucus and secretions within the uterine cavity). No observable changes in uterine size were recorded during an individual cycle.

Cul-de-sac: A small amount of fluid (estimated mean value 5–10 mL) demonstrated in the cul-de-sac.

Discussion

Interpretation of pelvic sonograms requires appreciation of the complex endocrine interactions which affect the female reproductive system. Since pelvic morphology changes in accordance with phases of the menstrual cycle, radiologists must become familiar with these phased alterations and the physiological environment of the ovaries and uterus they reflect.

The ovaries respond to two key hormones produced by the adenohypophysis: follicle-stimulating hormone (FSH) and luteinizing hormone (LH). Both hormones promote maturation of the primordial Graafian follicle. FSH causes growth of the ovum and its surrounding layers of granulosa and theca cells. LH, secreted by the pituitary at midcycle, completes follicle maturation, resulting in extrusion of the ovum. The other developing follicles then become atretic.

After the mature follicle has ruptured, the cells making up its rim become saturated with lipids, resulting in the characteristic yellow color: hence the name corpus luteum.

During the luteal phase, these cells, which are responsible for preovulation estrogen production, secrete increasing amounts of both estrogen and progesterone, which act as a negative feedback circuit on the pituitary, depressing FSH and LH production. The resulting decline in gonadotropin levels causes eventual involution of the corpus luteum, lowering blood progesterone and estrogen levels just prior to the onset on menses.

These ovarian hormones are also responsible for the uterine endometrial cycle. The rising estrogen levels in the first two weeks of the cycle cause stromal, glandular, and vascular proliferation. With the addition of progesterone in the latter part of the cycle, both hormones work synergistically to prepare the uterus for implantation. This results in the secretary endometrial phase, in which the mucosal glands swell with secretions and the blood vessels become engorged. Without implantation, estrogen and progesterone levels fall, causing shedding of the endometrium and resulting in menstruation (Figs 18.5 and 18.6).

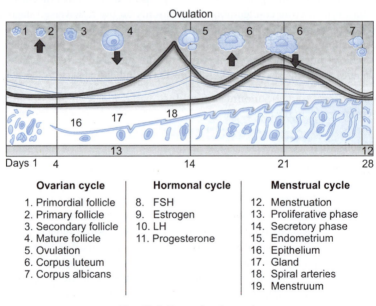

Ovarian cycle	Hormonal cycle	Menstrual cycle
1. Primordial follicle	8. FSH	12. Menstruation
2. Primary follicle	9. Estrogen	13. Proliferative phase
3. Secondary follicle	10. LH	14. Secretory phase
4. Mature follicle	11. Progesterone	15. Endometrium
5. Ovulation		16. Epithelium
6. Corpus luteum		17. Gland
7. Corpus albicans		18. Spiral arteries
		19. Menstruum

Fig. 18.5 Reproductive cycle

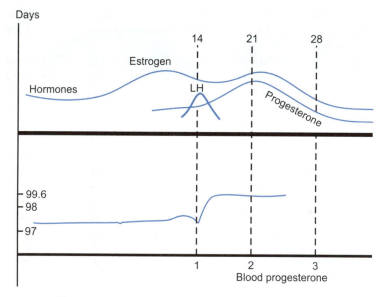

Fig. 18.6 Timing of the sequential sonograms in relation to basal body temperature and hormonal levels

This study discloses that normal hormonal influences on the female reproductive system may be associated with ultrasonographically observable effects. The ovaries display cystic elements which vary according to the stage of the menstrual cycle. At ovulation, the time of peak LH and FSH activity, ripening Graafian follicles are abundant. Ovarian cysts measuring approximately 1 cm in diameter were demonstrated most frequently at ovulation.

An additional ultrasonic manifestation of ovulation was small quantities of free peritoneal fluid in the cul-de-sac.

After ovulation, the corpus luteum develops and its hormonal functions dictate morphological changes in the ovaries and uterus. During the midluteal stage, larger ovarian cysts, approximately 2.0 cm in diameter, could be seen in cycles. These were considered corpora lutea, since they were not present at ovulation (Fig. 18.7).

Under the influence of the ovarian hormones of the luteal phase, the uterus displays a unique sonographic appearance resembling a "bull's-eye" on transverse images. The dense central echo from the uterine cavity is surrounded by a rim of relatively hypoechoic tissue. This may reflect vascular engorgement and glandular fluid in the thickened secretory endometrium.

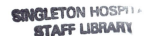

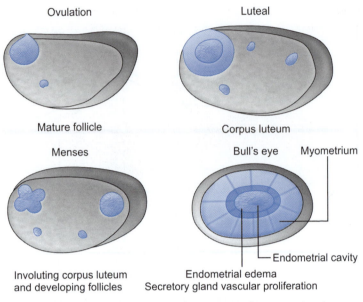

Ovulation

Luteal

Mature follicle

Corpus luteum

Menses

Bull's eye   Myometrium

Endometrial cavity

Involuting corpus luteum
and developing follicles

Endometrial edema
Secretory gland vascular proliferation

Fig. 18.7 Ultrasound study at three stages of menstrual cycle

The cyclic normal variations in the uterus and ovary should not be confused with gynecologic pathology. Physiological ovarian cysts may mimic small neoplasms or endometriosis. When free peritoneal fluid is present minimal ascites, inflammatory disease, and ectopic gestation enter the differential diagnosis. If the diagnosis is in doubt and the clinical condition permits, re-examination at a later date may help differentiate between pathological and physiological conditions. Pathological process may persist while physiological cysts and ovulatory fluid are transient phenomena which should not be seen if re-examination is performed at a subsequent phase of the menstrual cycle.

Acquired Uterine Disorders

Leiomyoma

They are usually multiple, and asymptomatic. The most frequent symptoms are pain and uterine bleeding. It can also cause infertility.

Myomas (Fibroids): They are submucus (least common), intramural (most common), subserous fibroids (pedunculated) and may simulate adnexal masses.

The classic ultrasound appearance of fibroid is hypoechoic, solid contour deforming mass in an enlarged inhomogenous uterus (Figs 18.8 and 18.9).

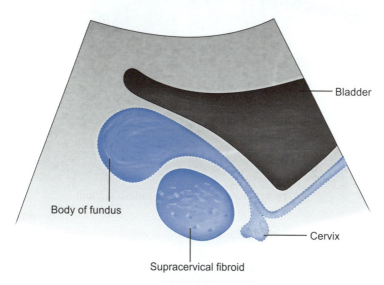

Fig. 18.8A Uterine fibroid (Longitudinal section)

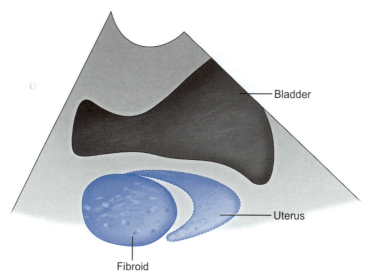

Fig. 18.8B Uterine fibroid (Transverse section)

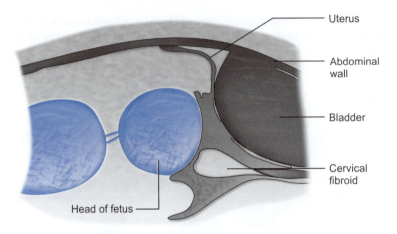

Fig. 18.9 Cervical fibroid (Longitudinal section)

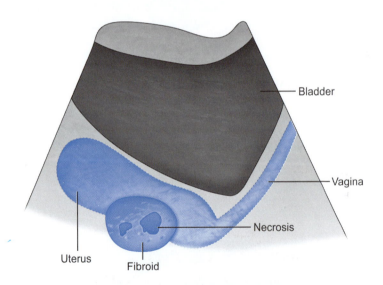

Fig. 18.10 Degenerating fibroid (Longitudinal section)

Myomas undergo a spectrum of secondary changes that include hyaline degeneration, fatty degeneration, calcification, hemorrhage and necrosis (Fig. 18.10).

Focal increased echogenicity occurs with fatty degeneration and calcification. The later may result in acoustic shadowing.

Degeneration or necrosis may result in decrease echogenecity and increased through transmission. Myoma also tends to become more hypoechoic during pregnancy.

In the gravid uterus, myometrial contractions (Braxton Hicks contraction) which last about few minutes to 1/2 hour and more, echogenic, should not be mistaken for myomas.

Myomas rarely develop in postmenopausal patients. Most tumors are stabilized or diminished in size after menopause. Postmenopausal increase in size of uterus may be due to sarcomatous changes.

The fundus of a retroverted uterus typically appears hypoechoic and a lobular contour is common so that the myomas are more difficult to diagnose in these patients.

Endometrial Polyps

Most polyps are symptomatic. The usual symptom is uterine bleeding. Sonographically polyps cause a prominent central uterine cavity echo. Polyps also cause uterine enlargement.

Endometrial Carcinoma

Postmenopausal bleeding is an important symptom. The ultrasound appearance is an enlarged uterus with irregular areas of low echoes and bizarre clusters of high intensity echoes (Fig. 18.11).

Endometrial carcinoma may obstruct the endometrial cavity resulting in hydrometra, pyometra or hematometra.

Leiomyosarcoma

It is the most frequent uterine sarcoma. Sonographically these tumors typically show large areas of degeneration, bizarre patches of high intensity echoes, invasion of surrounding structures and even distant metastases.

Cervical Carcinoma

This tumor occurs in woman between 45 and 55 years of age, factors causing development of carcinoma are multiparity, early onset of sexual relations, intercourse with uncircumcised males. The ultrasound scan usually shows a solid retrovesical mass. It is indistinguishable from a cervical myoma. There may be paracervical thickening of soft tissue, involvement of pelvic side walls and extension into bladder.

Cervical carcinoma also causes hydrometra, pyometra, hematometra.

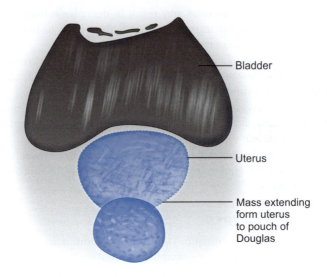

Fig. 18.11 Endometrial carcinoma (Transverse section)

Non-neoplastic Disorders

Endometrial Hyperplasia

This is due to unopposed estrogen stimulation. Endometrial hyperplasia is the most common cause of uterine bleeding. It occurs during the menstrual years as well as postmenopausal women. Ultrasound may demonstrate a prominent central uterine echo.

Adenomyosis

It is commonly seen in multiparus, between 30 and 40 years of age. Common symptoms are uterine bleeding and pain. Ultrasound appearance is irregular cystic spaces (fluid lakes) disrupt the homogeneity of uterine texture (Figs 18.12A and 18.12B).

Endometrioma

Apparently cystic mass free of internal echoes are visible in the region of ovaries, uterine ligaments, pelvic peritoneum (Figs 18.13 and 18.14).

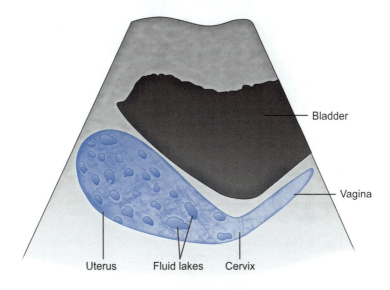

Fig. 18.12A Adenomyosis (Longitudinal section)

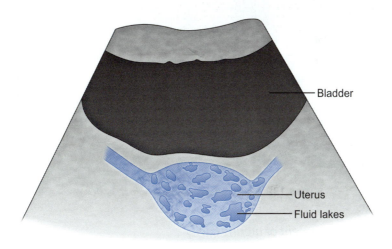

Fig. 18.12B Adenomyosis (Transverse section)

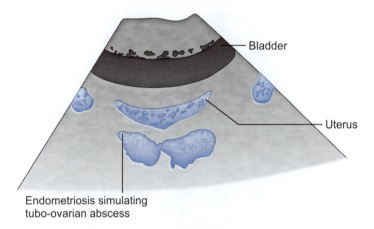

Fig. 18.13A Endometriosis simulating tubo-ovarian abscess
(Transverse section)

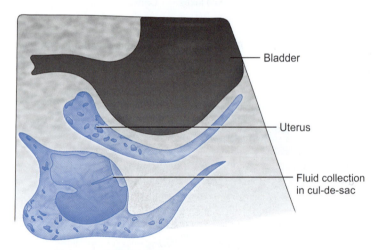

Fig. 18.13B Endometriosis (Longitudinal section)

Cystic enlargement of uterine cavity

- Hydrometra or pyometra
- Adenomyosis
- Degenerative fibroid
- Sarcomatous changes.

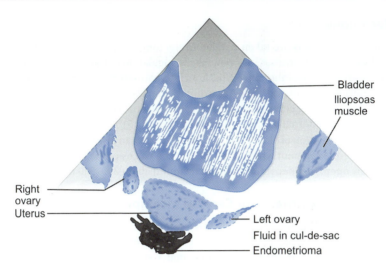

Fig. 18.14 Endometriosis simulating fluid in pouch of Douglas

Cervix

In pregnant uterus, the exact location of cervix and in particular the internal cervical os, is important. When a low lying placenta is detected, it allows for a determination of, whether the placenta covers the internal os termed a placenta previa. The overall length and width of the cervix is also helpful in diagnosing effacement due to either incompetent cervix or premature onset of labor.

To detect the endocervical canal as either a hyperechoic or hypoechoic band within cervix and define the internal os as either flat or very slightly funnel-shaped when the patient urinary bladder is moderately filled. The visualization varies with the stage of gestation, caused by difference in the size and position of fetus relative to cervix.

Prior to 20 weeks, the cervix could be clearly imaged in 100% patients, decreasing to 70% from 20–30 weeks and 18% between 30 weeks and term.

Incompetent Cervix

The classical obstetric history is painless cervical dilatation and recurrent second trimester loss, without associated bleeding or uterine contraction.

Dilated endocervical canal are visualized in three clinical situations: premature labor, inevitable abortion and incompetent cervix.

Technique

Longitudinal scans are taken parallel to the long axis of cervix, when the endocervical canal comes into view, slight angulation of transducer may be necessary to visualize the entire canal from internal os to external os. Following this transducer is rotated 90 degree to obtain transverse view of cervix. Using digital calipers, the cervical length, cervical width and width of cervical canal at the level of internal os can be measured (Fig. 18.15).

Over-distention of bladder should be avoided. It can distort the cervix and lower uterine segment which gives the cervix a close appearance when it is actually open. Bladder volume should be round about 300–500 mL.

Sonographic Criteria for Cervical Incompetence

During pregnancy in close cervix the endocervical canal appear either hyperechoic or occasionally hypoechoic band within the cervix. The lower uterine segment and cervix have a normal Y-shaped configuration. The internal os may vary from a flat to a slightly funnel-shaped.

Cervical Length

Over-distention of bladder compresses the anterior and posterior uterine wall leading to a false appearance of cervical elongation.

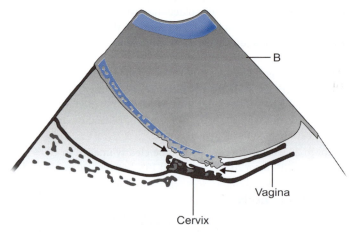

Fig. 18.15 Normal cervix—longitudinal midline scan of lower uterine segment performed through a distended urinary bladder (B). The cervix is defined in length (arrows) from external os to flattened internal os. Hypoechoic cervical canal is seen between two arrows

With transvaginal empty bladder technique, there may be false shortening because cervix is more vertically oriented.

In normal population mean cervical length is greater than 3 cm until about 32–34 weeks of gestation when gradual cervical effacement and shortening begins.

Progressive shortening of cervix is more significant than a single abnormal cervical length measurement.

In cervical incompetence the cervical length is less than 3 cm.

Cervical Width

On longitudinal scan, measurement of cervical width was made at the angle between the uterine cervix and body; at the point of greatest anteroposterior diameter.

In normal pregnancy cervical width is less than 2 cm in second trimester in pregnancy. Complicated by cervical incompetence the cervical width is more than 2 cm in second trimester.

Cervical Canal Width

Visualization of cervical canal allows the direct measurement of its width at the level of internal os.

In normal pregnancy cervical canal width is less than 8 mm and in cases of cervical incompetence it is more than 8 mm.

Bulging of the Membrane

Protrusion of membrane through the internal cervical os is the hallmark of the true incompetent cervix (Fig. 18.16) of the three measurements the width of the cervical canal is most reliable parameter to predict cervical incompetence. If dilatation of internal cervical os and bulging amnion are seen, the prognosis is unfavorable.

Cervical Cerclage

On sonographic examination of cervix, the suture appear as hyperechoic linear structures usually with acoustic shadowing. The anterior and posterior component of suture can be demonstrated in longitudinal and transverse views. The shadowing is more prominent in the region of surgical knot which is usually placed anteriorly.

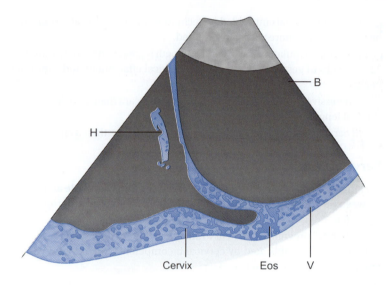

Fig. 18.16 Early herniation of membrane transabdominal longitudinal scan through a distended bladder, demonstrates, protrusion of membrane into proximal 2/3rd of cervical canal. The external os is closed.
Abbreviations: B, Bladder; H, Fetal head; V, Vagina; Eos, External os; Cervical canal width

Cervical Cancer

Etiology

Cervical epithelial neoplasia

- Cervical cancer can occur from child bearing age group to postmenopausal age groups
- Pap smear is positive
- Universal symptom is intermittent painless abnormal intermenstrual bleeding.

Ultrasound Findings

- Usually appears normal at early stage
- Enlarged lower uterine segment with distorted echogenicity of cervix area
- May see hematometra due to build up of fluid as a result of stenotic cervix

Intrauterine Devices

Localization

A number of intrauterine contraceptive devices (IUCD) can be recognized by 'longitudinal' sonogram (Figs 18.17A and B).

We see ultrasonographically:

- Shape of IUCD
- Entry and exit echo from IUCD
- Double line echoes
  - IUCD
  - Midline of uterine echo.

Coexistence of an IUCD and a gestational sac is not unusual. At a later stage of gestation, an IUCD may not be visible due to fetal parts.

Gestational Trophoblastic Disease

The condition is characterized by hydropic degeneration of villi resulting in vesicle formation.

Patient complains of vaginal bleeding (6–18 gestational weeks) ultrasonologically the uterus may be enlarged or normal in size. At low gain uterus appears empty. At high gain enlarged uterus is filled with "Snow flake appearance" (Fig. 18.18).

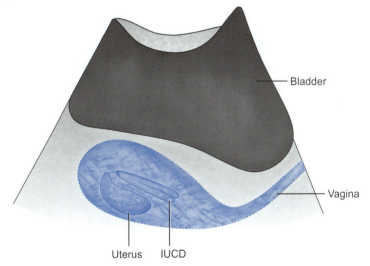

Fig. 18.17A Intrauterine device (Longitudinal section)

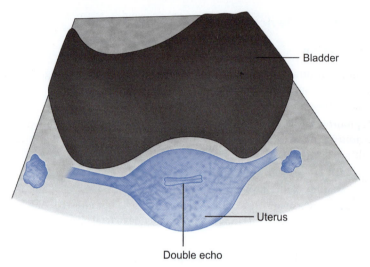

Fig. 18.17B Intrauterine device (Transverse section)

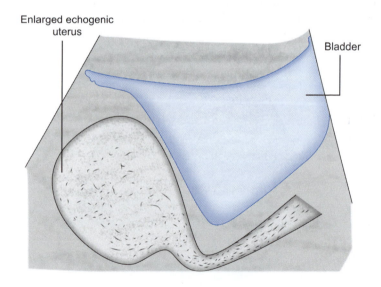

Fig. 18.18 Hydatidiform mole (Longitudinal section)

It is extremely important to do decreasing studies as well as increasing ones because if an identifiable fetal part is present within the uterus, it will resist being wiped out until after all placental/molar echoes have disappeared. This may dictate the method of uterine evacuation.

The earliest mole has very small vesicles, at approximately 8 weeks and these vesicles cannot be delineated by ultrasound. The resulting scan is therefore predominantly echogenic. By 18 weeks, the vesicles have a diameter of approximately 10 mm. These are easily identified by ultrasound. The varying degree of hemorrhage and necrosis give rise to varying degree of cystic changes within uterine content.

There are two types (pathological classification) of moles.

1. *True mole:* Only vesicles, no fetus or blood vessel seen. Trophoblastic proliferation is seen.
2. *Partial mole:* There are vesicles with fetus and blood vessels. Trophoblastic proliferation is very little.

    BHCG level increases in hydatidiform mole.

Differential Diagnosis

Hydropic degeneration of placenta. It tends to occur frequently after first trimester abortion. It is a partial mole. Degeneration of product of conception:

- Degenerating fibroid BHCG level is normal
- Pelvic masses simulating mole.
- Ovarian tumor
- Gut.

Choriocarcinoma with Pulmonary Metastases

A hydatidiform mole is potentially malignant condition and a choriocarcinoma arises in 1:40 moles, 1:15000 abortions. Pulmonary metastases are particularly common.

BHCG level increases in choriocarcinoma.

Causes of Uterine Enlargement

- Adenomyosis
- Hydatidiform mole
- Uterine fibroid
- Hydramnios
- Hydrocephalus

- Multiple pregnancy
- Endometrial polyp
- Recent abortion.

Abnormality of Uterine Shape

- Congenital anomaly
- Precocious puberty
- Retroposition
- Neoplasm benign or malignant.

Abnormality of Uterine Contour

- Endometriosis
- PID
- Neoplasm benign or malignant
- Postsurgery.

Abnormality in Uterine Texture

- Adenomyosis
- Hydatidiform mole
- Nabothian cyst
- Neoplasm—benign or malignant
- Pregnancy.

Prominence of Central Cavity Echo

- Early intrauterine pregnancy
- Ectopic pregnancy
- Endometrial hyperplasia
- Endometrial polyp
- Endometritis with PID
- Retained product of conception.

Ovaries

The ovaries are paired, almond-shaped organs approximately 2.5 cm long, weighing scarcely 1/4 of an oz. They are suspended by the broad ligaments on either side of the pelvis. Each ovary consists of two areas—a central medulla and an outer cortex. The medulla has many blood vessels in connective tissue.

The cortical portion contains the glandular tissue called follicles which are present in various stages of development. The ovaries are smooth and pink in the nulliparae but gray and puckered in the multiparae and elderly women due to the repeated discharge of the ova from its surface and the resultant scars. Eventually the ovaries become shrunken, wrinkled and atrophic.

These organs play a dominant role in determining sex drive, general health, femininity and moods.

At puberty, the ovaries are first stimulated by the pituitary gland to begin sexual maturation. Therefore, more than three decades they play a dynamic role in regulating the menstrual cycle and contributing to one of the basic materials of human life—the egg.

Actually, even before puberty each ovary contains approximately a million microscopic egg cells called oocytes. However, during the child-bearing years the ovary will produce about 400 eggs which are capable of fertilization (approximately one every 28 days) leaving a staggering reserve.

Selection of a particular egg for possible fertilization is not entirely understood; however, it is known that early in the menstrual cycle a minute amount of follicle stimulating hormone (FSH) is secreted. Extremely potent, this substance triggers a complex chain reaction in which several dormant egg cells are awakened and surrounded by a fluid-filled follicle. This double-like structure begins to expand and rapidly pushes toward the surface of the ovary.

Normally only one "bubble" succeeds in being released. However if two are released we have a case of multiple, nonidentical gestation. In approximately two week's time, the "bubble" appears as a blister about the size of a marble which protrudes from the outer surface of the ovary. It is at this time that another pituitary substance (luteinizing hormone LH) is secreted which causes the thin membrane covering the follicle to rupture. The contents spew out and the egg is carried along in the fluid into the funnel-shaped opening of the fallopian tube to await transport to the uterus in the event of successful fertilization. The size of the egg is so microscopic that it would take approximately 2 million eggs to fill thimble (Fig. 18.19).

The quality of the eggs is extremely important. Until approximately age 15, the potential of the eggs to achieve maturity and fertility is very poor. Even during the peak years (approximately 20–30) about 10–20% of the eggs usually fail to develop properly when fertilized and are rejected and either absorbed back into the body or aborted (blighted ovum).

As the female ages, the quality of the eggs declines and after age 40, chances of bearing a defective baby increase enormously, though the odds still favor a normal birth.

- Epithelium - a
- Tunica albuginea - b
- Capillaries in ovary - c
- Ovum - d
- Primordial follicle - e
- Secondary follicle - f
- Premature follicle - g
- Mature (Graafian) follicle - h
- Atretic follicle - i
- Ruptured follicle - j
- Discharged ovum - k
- Corpus hemorrhagicum - l
- Young corpus luteum - m
- Mature corpus luteum - n
- Corpus albicans - o
- Uterine tube - p
- Ovarian ligament - q
- Ovarian artery - r
- Ovarian vein - s
- Uterine artery - t

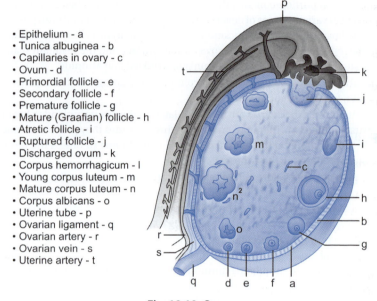

Fig. 18.19 Ovary

The ovaries produce the needed amount of estrogen to maintain proper function of the sexual organs. However, they also produce testosterone, the male hormone produced by the testicles. If this production is unbalanced, the result would be the appearance of masculinizing traits such as deepening voice and excessive growth of body hair. When the male-hormone production functions properly it is converted by the ovaries into estrogen.

Each month, the crater left by the ejected egg is filled with cells of a fatty, yellowish consistency. This becomes a new gland—the corpus luteum, which manufactures and secretes the hormone progesterone. Under the influence of progesterone the uterus prepares for pregnancy as stated before. If no pregnancy develops, the corpus luteum atrophies and dies.

In the presence of estrogen and progesterone imbalance, physical and emotional symptoms often appear, i.e. fluid retention, edema, irritability, nervousness and depression. A prescription of hormone therapy must then be instituted to achieve the proper balance.

The condition described above is called menopause and begins about age 40–50. The ovaries shrink back to prepuberty size and hormone production greatly decreases. Fatty deposits may appear through the body in the form of Dowager's hump and flabby breasts. Additionally, there is an increased susceptibility to fatty deposits within the arteries. Skin may become dry, muscles may stiffen and bones may become brittle.

The most serious threat to the ovaries is cancer. Early cancer of the ovary is often symptomless and beyond the range of a standard pelvic exam.

When the cancer is detectable as a mass, it is generally too late. Though this condition can strike at any age, its peak appearance is in the 45–60 age groups. Fortunately only 1 in 100 develop cancer of the ovary.

Follicular Maturation

Serial sonographic examinations can be used to determine

- Presence, number, size and growth of preovulatory follicles.
- Which ovary contains a mature follicle.
- Whether ovulation has occurred.

In general, the mature follicle at the time of ovulation in a patient undergoing spontaneous ovulation measures approximately 20 mm in average diameter. It has been noted that the follicles that range between 18 and 25 mm in diameter have the greatest number of granulosa cells, and indication of follicular maturity (Fig. 18.20).

Most frequently corpus luteum can be distinguished from a developing follicle by its irregular wall and internal echoes.

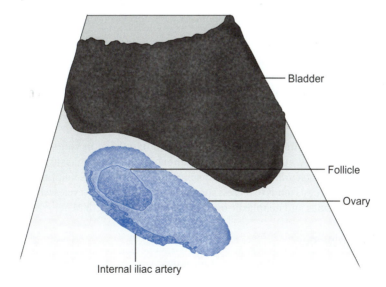

Fig. 18.20 Follicular development (Longitudinal section)

In most patients, a small amount of fluid (5–10 mL) can be seen in cul-de-sac immediately after ovulation occurs. The wall of follicle becomes noticeably irregular.

Patients, who are candidates for *in vitro* fertilization and embryo transfer, are examined daily being approximately 5 days prior to anticipated date of ovulation. The size of each ovarian follicle is noted on each examination. The average dimension of the follicle in transverse and anteroposterior or long axis is utilized.

Serial sonographic examinations also have a very important role in the patients who undergo ovulation induction therapy. Follicles in patients with polycystic ovaries that undergo hormonal induction are larger than in patient with nonstimulated cycle. A mature follicle in stimulated patient usually ranges from 25–35 mm in greatest dimension.

Ovarian Mass

Cystic Adnexal Masses

Cystic masses demonstrate very even texture (homogenous mass). Through transmission is good (Low attenuation of fluid suspension). Distal acoustic enhancement.

Several types of adnexal masses exhibit a cystic texture:
- Physiological ovarian cyst
- Benign cyst adenoma
- Paraovarian cysts
- Hydrosalpinges
- Endometriomas
- Tubo-ovarian mass.

Physiological Ovarian Cysts

They are most common in infant female and in woman in child bearing age group. They appear as rounded anechoic adnexal masses. Serial evaluation of such unilocular cysts by sonography may be quite helpful, since physiological cysts tends to regress spontaneously over several cycles whereas endometriomas and neoplastic ovarian cystic do not (Fig. 18.21).

Hydrosalpinges

They tend to be fusiform in shape whereas ovarian cysts are usually spherical. It is anechoic (Fig. 18.22).

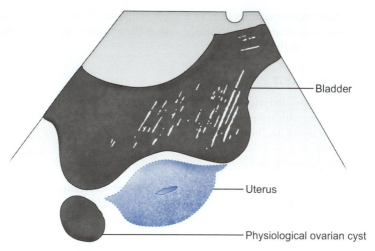

Fig. 18.21 Physiological ovarian cyst (Transverse section)

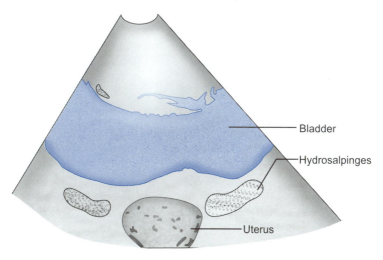

Fig. 18.22 Hydrosalpinges (Transverse section)

Tubo-ovarian Abscess

It results from chronic pelvic inflammatory disease. These masses tend to have a layer of low level echoes which represent pus within the tubo-ovarian abscess. Patients with hydrosalpinx or tubo-ovarian abscess may present with right upper quadrant pain as a result of infected fluid tracking up the right paracolic recess to localize in the subhepatic and perihepatic space (Fitz Hugh Curtis syndrome).

Ovarian Abscess

They are associated with intrauterine contraceptive device. These abscesses are localized within corpus luteum. They arise from low grade endometritis produced by IUCD. These are anechoic masses.

Para-ovarian Cysts

They are remnants of Wolffian duct system. These masses range from 2–3 cm. They do not demonstrate cystic regression like physiological ovarian cyst.

Endometrioma

They are apparently cystic mass free of echoes (Fig. 18.23).

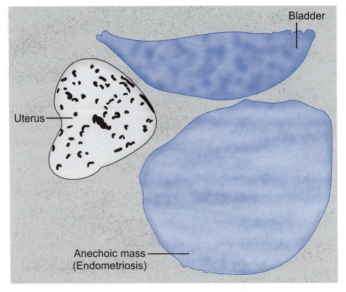

Fig. 18.23 Endometriosis simulating multilocular cystadenoma

Complex Predominently Cystic Masses

These masses are predominently cystic masses, that contain septa, internal contents or solid material.

They are cystadenoma, dermoid cyst and tubo-ovarian abscesses.

Cystadenoma

These are large cystic masses with internal septa. Usually patients with these types of tumor are postmenopausal. They present progressive abdominal enlargement for several months. More solid and irregular areas within the mass, the more likely is tumor malignant. Malignancy can also be inferred when ascitis is associated with the mass (Fig. 18.24).

Once a mass of this variety is encountered one should examine pericolic recesses, subhepatic space and cul-de-sac for the presence of ascites.

Liver for the presence of hepatic metastases should be seen. These are mostly hypoechoic masses or anechoic masses with irregular border.

Dermoid Cyst

Dermoid cysts are classically highly echogenic. Echogenic mass seen within this cyst, however, is highly suggestive of dermoid.

When a dermoid is purely cystic or contains some internal debris, it is indistinguishable from an endometrioma, cystadenoma, hemorrhagic ovarian cysts.

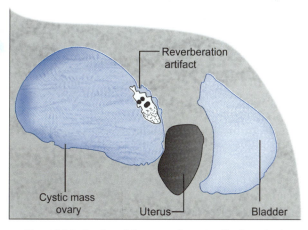

Fig. 18.24 Cystic pelvic tumor (Longitudinal section)

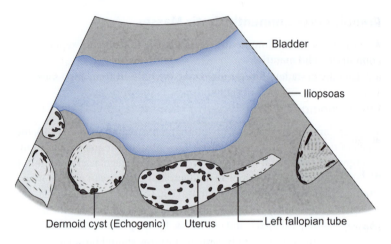

Fig. 18.25 Echogenic dermoid cyst (Transverse section)

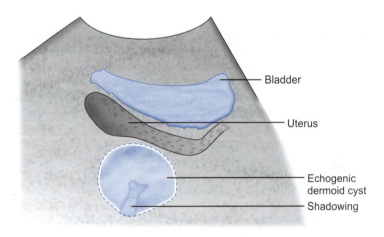

Fig. 18.26 Dermoid cyst with calcification (Longitudinal section)

The presence of highly echogenic mass within a cystic area or a presence of an echogenic mass that feels cystic is highly suggestive of dermoid (Fig. 18.25).

Shadowing is seen from echogenic mass. This could be due to calcified element-tooth (Fig. 18.26).

Predominently Solid Masses

A complex predominently solid mass consists primarily of soft tissue components or contain echogenic internal material such as sebum within a dermoid cyst or numerous floating cells contained within the mass (Figs 18.27 and 18.28). This type of mass can also result from cystic degeneration within a solid mass such as characteristically found in granulosa cell tumor.

The most common types of complex predominantly solid ovarian masses are germ cells tumor or ovarian neoplasm.

Solid Ovarian Tumors

The solid tumors of ovary are rare.

Meigs Syndrome

Ovarian fibroma, ascites and pleural effusion (Fig. 18.29). Sonographic mimic of ovarian masses:

- Fluid-filled loops of bowel
- Para-ovarian cyst
- Multiple endometrioma
- Hematoma.

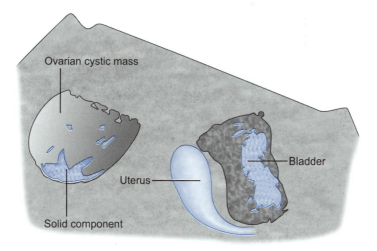

Fig. 18.27 Mixed pelvic tumor

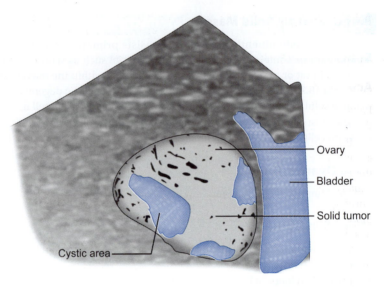

Fig. 18.28 Cystadenocarcinoma of ovary (Longitudinal section)

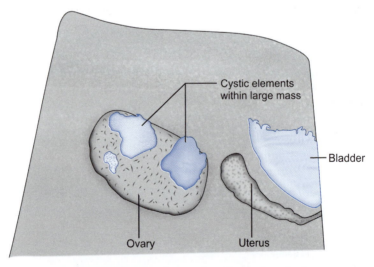

Fig. 18.29 Fibroma of ovary (Longitudinal section)

PELVIC INFLAMMATORY DISEASES

Sonographic Evaluation of Pelvic Infections

Acute Pelvic Inflammatory Disease

Pelvic inflammatory disease results from ascending infection, traveling through endometrium, salpinges and into the peritoneum.

If pelvic inflammatory disease is not promptly and adequately treated, adhesions may obstruct the fallopian tube and lead to a pyosalpinx. If the ovary is also involved in the infection tubo ovarian abscess may form, usually bilateral. Pelvic peritonitis and pelvic abscess may also develop when purulent material spills from fallopian tubes. Rupture of abscess may lead to more extensive abscess formation often presenting in the right subphrenic or subhepatic space.

Tubo-ovarian abscess are associated with the findings of fever, purulent discharge and leukocytosis which are not present in necrotic tumors (Figs 18.30 and 18.31).

Sonography

Pyosalpinx and tubo-ovarian abscess are characteristically tubular adnexal masses (Figs 18.32A and B).

There may be typical sonographic features of fluid collections. Abscess may also have thick and irregular or shaggy wall; or may contain echoes or fluid levels representing the layering of purulent debris.

Free pelvic fluid may indicate peritonitis. If free fluid becomes loculated an abscess may form (commonly in cul-de-sac).

Differential Diagnosis

Cystic mass with septation and debris (multilocular lesion):
- Cystadenoma of ovary
- Cystadenocarcinoma
- Tubo-ovarian abscess
- Endometriosis
- Ectopic pregnancy.

Bilateral Adnexal Masses

- Bilateral ovarian cysts
- Bilateral tubo-ovarian abscesses
- Endometriosis.

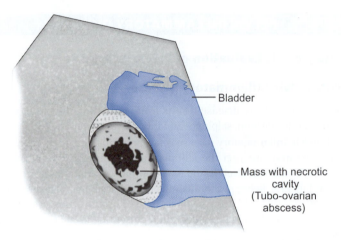

Fig. 18.30A Tubo-ovarian abscesses (Transverse section)

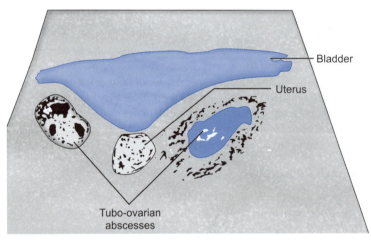

Fig. 18.30B Tubo-ovarian abscesses (Longitudinal section)

Chronic Pelvic Inflammatory Disease

The term chronic pelvic inflammatory disease refers to the residue of acute infection and to subacute reinfection of previous acute pelvic inflammatory disease.

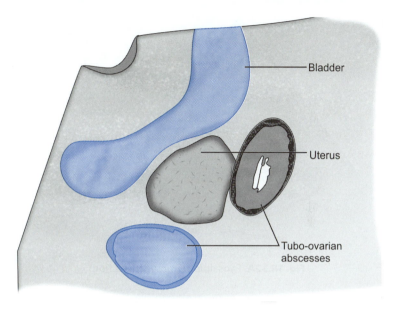

Fig. 18.31A Tubo-ovarian abscesses (Transverse section)

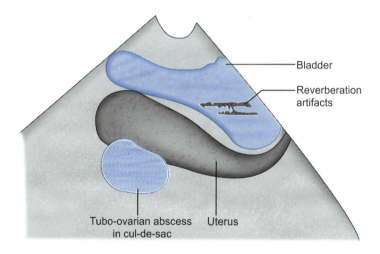

Fig. 18.31B Tubo-ovarian abscesses (Longitudinal section)

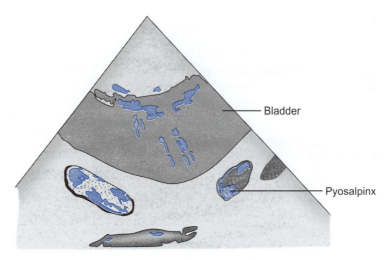

Fig. 18.32A Pyosalpinx (Transverse section)

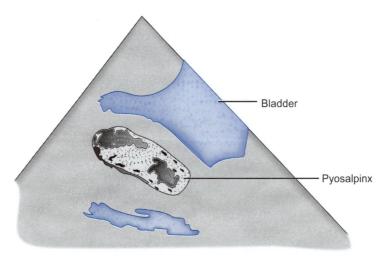

Fig. 18.32B Pyosalpinx (Longitudinal section)

Sonography

Echogenicity of uterus and endometrial cavity returns to normal from indefinite uterus of acute pelvic inflammation. Complex pattern of pelvic fluid loculations are not visible in cul-de-sac region because of adhesion.

D/D   (Bilateral cystic septate lesions).
       Bilateral necrotic tumors
       Multilocular cystadenoma of ovaries.

The main causes of pelvic inflammatory diseases are:

- Ascending   (Venereal)
                      IUCD
- Perforation   Periappendicular abscess
                      IUCD perforates through uterine wall.
- Surgery after cesarean section.

19

Infertility

Infertility is defined as inability to conceive a wanted child after 12 months of unprotected intercourse. Ultrasound plays an integral and an indispensable part.

Conditions in which ultrasound may contribute to the diagnosis of infertility.

1. Uterine factors
   a. Congenital uterine abnormalities
   b. Uterine fibroid
2. Fallopian tubes obstructions
   a. Ectopic pregnancy
   b. Endometriosis
   c. Pelvic inflammatory disease
3. Ovarian factor
   a. Polycystic ovaries (PCO)
   b. Hypothalamic amenorrhea
   c. Luteinized unruptured follicle (LUF).

Uterine Factors

Congenital Anomalies

Congenital anomalies of uterus are common with early fetal wastage.

Uterus didelphys: Slow transverse scanning will reveal two endometrial cavities. This finding can be confirmed by sagittal scanning which will demonstrate the endometrial echoes (echogenic) separated by myometrium (relative hypoechoic). Ultrasound determines the side on which ovulation is taking place.

Bicornuate uterus (two horn and a single cervix) may be complete, partial or arcuate. This rarely causes fetal wastage. Those with unicornuate may be fertile. Patients with septate uterus are often infertile or suffer early fetal wastage.

Fibroids

Uterine fibroids have been associated with infertility and early fetal loss. They vary in size and may grow very large. They may be submucous, intramural subserous or pedunculated. Ultrasound study reveals irregular uterine contour, a focal mass either hypoechoic or hyperechoic and in some uterine enlargement, GnRH agonists have been used in the treatment of patients of fibroid. GnRH causes decrease in the size of uterine fibroid. This can be confirmed by follow-up study by ultrasound.

Fallopian Tubes Obstruction

Ectopic Pregnancy

The trial of empty uterus, free fluid and adnexal mass coupled with positive pregnancy test should alert the possibility of ectopic pregnancy.

A diagnosis can be made by the demonstration of live ectopic pregnancy (cardiac pulsations visible). Sometime only a complex adnexal mass is visible. In such cases, color Doppler study reveal trophoblastic flow pattern "ring of fire" appearance [by transvaginal scan (TVS) study].

Endometriosis

Patient normally complains with infertility dysmenorrhea and dyspareunia. It is suggested that an ovulatory disorder is the cause of infertility in endometriosis. Ultrasound study shows a well-defined hypoechoic mass with internal echoes.

Pelvic Inflammatory Disease

Predisposing factors for pelvic inflammatory disease (PID) include:
- Gonococcal salpingitis
- Multiple sexual partners
- Use of intrauterine device.

Normally, patient complains of lower abdominal pain, purulent discharge and fever.

Ultrasound Findings

- Early phase—uterus may be enlarged with indistinct margin. There may be mild adnexal enlargement.

- Severe phase—ill-defined areas of decreased echogenicity (cystic or solid in appearance) may be seen. It may be associated with fluid in cul-de-sac.
- Finally frank abscess may develop.

Differential Diagnosis

- Hematoma
- Endometriosis
- Ectopic pregnancy.

Ovarian Factor

Polycystic Ovaries

It is an endocrine abnormality resulting from chronic anovulation. The most common symptoms are amenorrhea, hirsutism, obesity and infertility.

The correct diagnosis of PCO is important not only for diagnosing a cause of infertility but it may also be life saving as patient with elevated estrogen have a significant increased risk of endometrial carcinoma and possible ovarian malignancy.

Ultrasound Examination

Ovarian size is increased. Ovary may be hypoechoic. Multiple cysts of different sizes are present in ovary (Fig. 19.1).

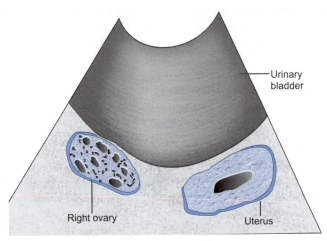

Fig. 19.1 Polycystic ovary disease

One very useful finding in identifying woman with PCO is in assessment of endometrial echo thickness.

Treatment of PCO may be initiated with a trial of clomiphene citrate (CC), ultrasound is often performed near the expected mid cycle (after a progestran induced withdrawal bleed).

If ovulation fails to occur then hCG may be added mid cycle to induce ovulation.

Hypothalamic Amenorrhea

There is another group of cystic ovarian disease entities—hypothalamic amenorrhea.

Patient who developed amenorrhea secondary to weight loss, extensive exercise, lactation, after cessation of birth control pills.

Ultrasound Findings

The cysts are most often circumferentially oriented in the ovary. The type of cyst almost invariably have low estrogen level.

Luteinized Unruptured Follicle

In patient with luteinized unruptured follicle (LUF), the follicle does not rupture on expected day (in mid day of cycle) and achieves a size much larger than normal preovulatory size of 2 cm.

Ultrasound (with TVS) one can observe failure of follicle to deflate and absence of intraperitoneal fluid associated with ovulation (Fig. 19.2).

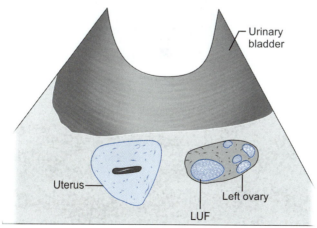

Fig. 19.2 Luteinized unruptured follicle (LUF)

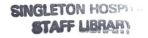

Follicular Monitoring

Ultrasound has a vital role in depicting follicular development in infertility patients. The maturity of oocyte is only indirectly inferred by the size of follicle. The sonographic information can be coupled with serum estradiol values to provide an accurate assessment of the presence or absence of mature follicles.

Some infertility specialists describe an abnormality in ovulation called Luteinized unruptured follicle (LUF) syndrome as a cause of unexplained infertility. In LUF, there is failure of extrusion of the oocyte which remains trapped within the follicle. With ultrasound (TVS) one can observe failure of the follicle to deflate and the absence of intraperitoneal fluid associated with ovulation.

Spontaneous Ovulation

When menarche begins approximately 2,00,000 primary oocyte remain per ovary. During the child bearing years approximate 200 oocytes will be ovulated.

Maturation of the oocyte and follicle is responsive primarily to changes in follicle stimulating hormone (FSH), luteinizing hormone (LH) and circulating levels of estrogen (E_2).

Beginning with normal cycle there is usually one or sometimes two dominant follicles are seen. TVS can depict the developing follicles starting when they measure between 3 and 5 mm (Fig. 19.3).

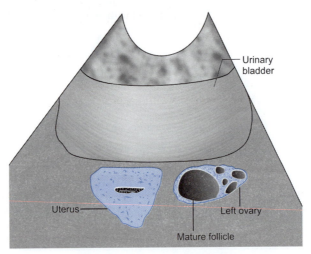

Fig. 19.3 Normal mature follicle

As the follicle matures, more fluid is elaborated into its center and the number of granulosa cells lining the inner wall of follicle increases. The oocyte which is less than a tenth of a millimeter, is surrounded by a cluster of granulosa cells. This complex is termed the cumulus oophorus. It measures approximately 1 mm. Sometime it can be seen in follicle with TVS. Immediately before ovulation the cumulus separates from the wall and floats freely in the center of follicle.

By day 5-7 of menstrual cycle (Early follicular phase), several recruited follicles may be seen. At this time process of dominance begins.

By day 8-12 of menstrual cycle (late follicular phase) the dominant follicle can be detected. Other follicles will begin to diminish in size. The non-dominant follicles usually do not exceed 1.4 cm in diameter. In 5-10% of cycles two dominant follicle may be seen.

From 4 to 5 days before ovulation growth of the dominant follicle is linear, increasing by 2-3 mm per day. Maximum mean diameter is 20-24 mm with a range of 18-24 mm.

95% of measurable serum E_2 in a normal cycle is elaborated by dominant follicle. The E_2 level usually peaks 24-36 hours before ovulation. This rise in E_2 causes an LH surge. The LH surge usually begins 28-36 hours before follicular rupture.

Intrafollicular echoes may be observed (by TVS) with mature follicle probably arising from clusters of granulosa cells that sheer off the wall near the time of ovulation.

After ovulation (early luteal phase), the follicular wall becomes irregular (follicle deflated). The fresh corpus (early luteal phase) usually appear as hypoechoic structure with irregular wall. It may contain some internal echoes corresponding to hemorrhage.

As corpus luteum develops 4-8 days after ovulation (mid luteal phase) it appear as echogenic structure of approximately 15 mm. Its wall is thickened by process of luteinization.

It is normal to have approximately 1-3 mL of fluid in cul-de-sac throughout the cycle. When ovulation occurs there is typically 4-5 mL of fluid in cul-de-sac.

Induced Ovulation

In patients whose infertility can be attributed to an ovulation abnormality, ovulation induction is indicated. Ovulation induction is also used in *in vitro* fertilization embryo transfer (IVF-ET), to increase the number of oocytes aspirated which in turn increase the number of fertilized conception, that may be transferred hereby increasing the chance of pregnancy.

Two medication most commonly used for ovulating induction are clomiphene citrate (CC) and human menopausal gonadotropin (hMG).

Patient undergoing ovulation study are usually examined every other day beginning between day 7 and 9. For patient undergoing IVF-ET patient begin to be examined by TVS earlier in their cycles and usually daily in an attempt to carefully monitor their follicular development.

Clomiphene citrate (CC) is considered as estrogen antagonist and exerts its effects by binding estrogen receptor sites in the pituitary and hypothalamus. This leads to increased FSH secretion by pituitary thereby recruiting more synchronous follicles. Some patients are given human chorionic gonadotropin (hCG) once follicle reaches 15 mm to 18 mm in size to induce final follicular and oocyte maturation. Follicular development with CC can be different than that observed in spontaneous cycle. Each follicle seems to develop at an individual rate and at time may be accelerated or slowed down. Therefore, the largest follicle on a giving date may not be the same 2 days later and may not even be the one that is most mature. Correlation of E_2 and follicle sizes are poor. Maximum preovulatory diameter can range from 19 to 24 mm (Fig. 19.4).

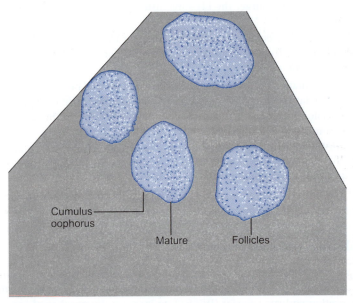

Fig. 19.4 Multiple mature follicles. Ovulation induction with clomid

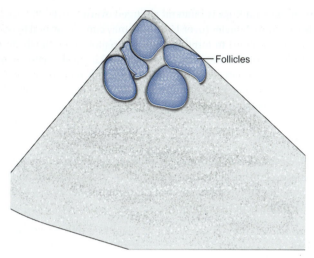

Fig. 19.5   Multiple follicles. Ovulation induction with hMG

Treatment with hMG does not require an intact hypothalamus or pituitary. The response to endogenous gonadotropins is to develop a small number of large follicles. The growth rate and E_2 secretion are linear correlate well and are of equal predictive value. A high pregnancy rate is achieved in this group (Fig. 19.5).

After induced ovulation stimulated follicle usually undergo regression but may persist and enlarge over the reminder of cycle "physiological ovarian cyst over 3 cm".

In vitro fertilization follicles are typically aspirated when they reach 15–18 mm in average dimension and when there is evidence of estradiol values of mature follicle (approximately 400 pg/mL/mature follicle). Higher pregnancy rate is achieved in those patient whose mature follicle demonstrates intrafollicular echoes (clumps of granulosa cells).

Ovarian Hyperstimulation Syndrome

Most patients who undergo ovulation induction ranging from mild abdominal discomfort, severe circulatory compromise and electrolyte imbalance (ascites, pleural effusion). The enlarged ovaries may be prone to torsion. The symptoms associated with ovarian hyperstimulation syndrome (OHSS) usually begin 5–8 days after hCG is given or in patient who get pregnant.

Sonographic findings is bilateral enlarged ovaries (over 10 cm), having multiple immature follicles (over 15 mm). It may contain several hypoechoic areas, may correspond to atretic follicles or region of hemorrhage within ovaries. Color Doppler sonography may be useful in the detection of ovarian torsion. Torsion may affect one arterial blood supply more than other (ovary has dual blood supply one from uterine artery, the other coursing through the infundibulopelvic ligament).

Endometrium

There is a clear association of sonographic texture of the endometrium and circulating levels of estrogen and progesterone. In spontaneous and induced cycles, the sonographic appearance of the endometrium varies according to its specific phase of development.

Menstrual phase: The endometrium appears as a thin broken echogenic interphase.

Proliferative phase: It thickens and becomes isoechoic, measuring 3–5 mm in anteroposterior width. It is hypoechogenic. It is due to relatively orderly organization of the glandular elements within the endometrium.

Preovulatory phase: As ovulation approaches, the endometrium becomes more echogenic. This is due to development of secretion within the endometrial glands and the numerous interfaces that arise from distended and tortuous glands.

Periovulatory period: There is usually a hypoechoic area within the inner endometrium. It represents edema of compactum layer.

Secretory phase: The endometrium achieves its greatest thickness (between 6 and 12 mm) and echogenicity.

In addition to the echogenic endometrium, a hypoechoic band beneath the endometrium can be identified probably arising from the inner layer of myometrium.

In only small number of cases (4%), the measurement of endometrial thickness is not possible.

Medication used for ovulation induction may alter the development of endometrium, has been shown sonographically. Patient treated with clomid citrate show a mean endometrial thickness of 2.9 mm compared with 3.2 mm for patient treated with hMG and 3.1 mm for controls. In controls, the maximum mean endometrial thickness was 4.9 mm in secretory phase of cycle.

The conception is unlikely in endometria that measures less than 13 mm (including both layers), 11 days after ovulation.

Role of Color Doppler in Infertility

The advent of transvaginal color Doppler sonography has added a new dimension to the diagnosis and treatment of infertile female.

Study of Menstrual Cycle by Color Doppler

It is very important to study the whole of menstrual cycle by transvaginal color Doppler during the evaluation of infertility. It provides vital information about follicular dynamics like blood flow to growing follicle, the vascular supply of endometrium and corpus luteum visualization which are very important for a successful outcome in terms of pregnancy.

Changes in the Ovary

Both ovaries measure about 2.2–5.5 cm in length, 1.5–2 cm in width and 1.5–3 cm in depth. The ovaries are recognized by the presence of follicles of different sizes. The blood supply is by ovarian artery and ovarian branch of uterine artery. The primary and secondary branches of ovarian artery grow alongwith the development of dominant follicle, which can be recognized by TVS color Doppler by 8 or 10 day of cycle by a ring of angiogenesis around it, whereas other follicle do not demonstrate this. The vessels around dominant follicle become more abundant and prominent as the follicle grow to 20–24 mm.

The phases are described as:

   I. Early follicular (day 5–7)

  II. Late follicular (day 11–13)

 III. Early luteal (day 15–17)

 IV. Late luteal (day 26–28).

Index values: These are high in early part of menstrual cycle and fall as ovulation approaches.

- RI in early proliferative phase is – 0.54 +/–0.04
- RI in late follicular phase before ovulation (LH peak) – 0.44 +/–0.04.
- This is the best time for administration of surrogate hCG.
- RI in mid luteal phase (lowest) – 0.42 +/–0.06.
- RI in late luteal phase shows higher vascular resistance – 0.50 +/–0.04.

Corpus Luteum

The dominant ovary corpus luteum show a low impedance wave form with RI of 0.39–0.49 characteristic of blood flow in early pregnancy. The contralateral ovary show a high impedance flow with RI of 0.69–1.00 characteristic of non-dominant ovary.

In patient with corpus luteum deficiency the vascularity is not optimal and the RI is raised to around 0.59. With decreased diastolic flowed. RI of >0.5 is associated with nonviable outcome.

Secretory Changes in the Endometrium

Michael Applebaum divided the endometrium into 4 zones. According to him, no pregnancy was reported in IVF patients unless vascularity was demonstrated in zone III or IV prior to transfer.

CHAPTER 20

Obstetrics

Introduction to Obstetrical Ultrasound

There are three major stages in the prenatal period:
1. Ovum
2. Embryonic
3. Fetal.

While diagnostic ultrasound can effectively image the embryonic and fetal stages, due to the size of the conceptus and the resolution limits of currently available equipment, though it cannot be imaged, the ovum should be understood.

Ovum Stage

Assuming a 29-day cycle, on approximately the 10–14th day after the beginning of the LMP, a mature follicle ruptures and leaves the ovary, traveling into the Fallopian tube. Sperm deposited during this time (within the vagina) travel through the cervix, into the uterus and out into the Fallopian tube.

Fertilization occurs in the distal portion of the tube and the now fertilized ovum (zygote) continues its journey to the site of implantation, the fundus of the uterus.

In early embryonic development it is difficult to differentiate the rapidly multiplying cells, but at about 16 days the embryo shows a primitive streak from with 3 types of tissues develop: an outer layer of ectoderm a middle layer or mesoderm and an internal layer or endoderm. The product of conception is called an embryo until the 9th week, from that time until delivery it is called a fetus.

As the embryo continues to grow, definite structures develop from the three germ cell layers:
1. *Ectoderm:* Produces skin, brain tissue, nervous system and certain cutaneous structure.

2. *Mesoderm:* Yields muscle and circulatory organs, the reproductive system and connective tissue of other organs.
3. *Endoderm:* Provides the digestive tract and organs connected with it such as the liver, pancreas and lungs.

Approximately 7–9 days after ovulation the fertilized egg implants itself into the uterus. The site of this implantation process is referred to as its nidation.

The lining of the uterus or endometrium has been preparing for this event and is in its progestational or secretory phase, ready to receive the new life on this, the 21st–23rd days of the cycle.

The outside of the fertilized egg is surrounded by a single layer of ectodermic cells called chorion. Soon after the embryo buries itself in the endometrium, many small villi or fingers of tissue reach out to obtain nourishment for the embryo. These fingers are called trophoblasts and are nourishing cells that form the fetal part of the placenta. Wherever trophoblasts grow into the basal endometrium they will eventually take nourishment from the maternal blood and become fastening villi as well as nourishing ones. The villi on the side of the embryonic sac which extends into the uterine cavity seen atrophy and are called chorion laeve.

With pregnancy, the uterine lining takes on a new morphology called the decidua (meaning something to be cast off or discarded). For descriptive purposes, the decidua are divided into three categories:
1. Decidua basalis
2. Decidua capsularis
3. Decidua vera or parietalis.

The endometrial layer where the trophoblasts bury themselves is called the decidua basalis and it is this layer which fuses with the trophoblasts to form the maternal portion of the placenta. As the embryo grows within the uterus it is first covered by the decidua capsularis. At about 3 months the embryo and its coverings fill the uterus and are now in approximation with the other layer, the decidua vera or parietalis (Fig. 20.1).

Embryonic Stage

This occurs as soon as the fertilized ovum attaches to the maternal uterine wall and lasts until the 8–9th week of uterine life. By the end of this period the embryo will be almost 4 cm long and will weigh about 2/3rd of an ounce. It is at this time that positive signs of fetal life can easily be elicited. This may be observed as real-time cardiac motion or audible fetal heart tones recorded by a Doppler device.

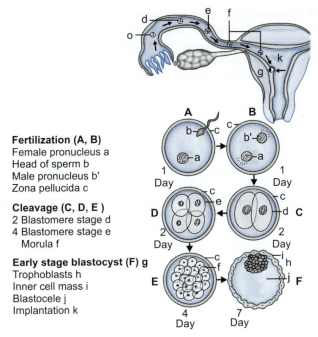

Fertilization (A, B)
Female pronucleus a
Head of sperm b
Male pronucleus b'
Zona pellucida c

Cleavage (C, D, E)
2 Blastomere stage d
4 Blastomere stage e
  Morula f

Early stage blastocyst (F) g
Trophoblasts h
Inner cell mass i
Blastocele j
Implantation k

Fig. 20.1 Development of the embryo (part I)

This is a period of rapid growth and includes the beginnings of the three structures essential for the protection and nourishment of the embryo:

1. Placenta
2. Umbilical cord
3. Amniotic sac.

The placenta develops at the point of implantation of the ovum to the uterine wall. It is a vascular organ which contains channels for the exchange of fluids.

The incoming maternal blood contains nourishment, oxygen, antigens and hormones—whereas the outgoing blood essentially contains waste products. At term, the placenta (often referred to as the after birth) is cast off by the uterus after the fetus is expelled. Its appearance at that time is of a round, flattened organ looking very much like a pancake (for which it is named). Expelled placenta vary in size but are generally about 20 cm in diameters and 3 cm thick. The ultrasonic appearance of the placenta *in utero* is quite different. During its intrauterine stage the placenta is filled with blood and at various sites of its attachment its thickness may vary from 2–6 cm.

The fetal membranes extend from the margins of the placenta. The layer closest to the uterus is called the chorion and represents the outside layer of the original egg and the chorionic laeve. A thin, inner layer of tissue called the amnion encloses the embryo and continues downward to also cover the umbilical cord. The amnion secretes a clear alkaline liquid called amniotic fluid. The amniotic sac is a nonvascular, transparent membrane which completely encases the embryo except at the point where the umbilical cord projects itself into the placenta and the uterine wall, acts as a buffer against shocks, an insulator against loud noises, promotes warmth and serves as a magnificent 'water bed' for the developing fetus.

The umbilical cord is a tube-like, vascular organ connecting the placenta to the abdominal wall of the embryo. It is generally 50 cm in length and contains two arteries and the larger umbilical vein. Nourishment is carried by way of the umbilical vein from the placenta to the fetus and the waste products from the fetus are carried back through the two arteries to the placenta. The flexibility of the cord permits considerable activity during the fetal stage making it possible occasionally for a fetus to become entangled in the cord so that a true knot forms. It is even possible for the cord to become drapped around the baby's body or neck so tightly as to cut off circulation (Fig. 20.2).

Fetal Stage

At about the 9th to 10th week of uterine life the fetal head and thorax distance can be visualized and measured ultrasonically. This crown-rump length of the fetus is the most accurate indicator of fetal age (Figs 20.3 and 20.4). The fetus is now about 5–6 cm long weighing only 1 ounce, but it has travelled very far along the road to birth and is essentially a miniature human—with heart, lung, brain, spinal cord, sensory organs, face and even stubby fingers and toes. Over the remaining fetal period it will continue to grow and refine its structures, but the major activity of the fetus will be to learn to use and coordinate all the intricate and delicate equipment it has been building during the embryonic stage. Some highlights of fetal development over the next 7 months are:

3rd month: Fetal activity increases. Respiratory-like movements have been reported and urea can be detected in the amniotic fluid, indicating kidney function.

4th month: Now about 18 cm long, the fetus has reached about half its height at birth. The entire reproductive system has been formed and a whole range of activities have developed such as thumb sucking and hiccuping. All the reflexes found in a normal newborn are present except for vocal responses and functional respiration.

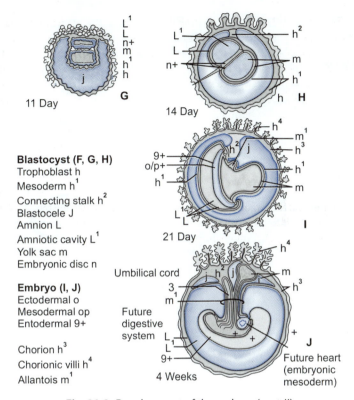

Fig. 20.2 Development of the embryo (part-II)

5th month: Now about 24 cm long, the fetus weights approximately 1 lb. Its movements can be felt by the mother as real kicks. Because it is floating around in the amniotic sac, it has marvelous ease and can assume a variety of movements and positions. In fact some fetuses are noticeably active 75% of the time.

6th month: Fetal breathing motions (30–100/min) may be observed with a real-time scanner, from this stage and through term.

7th month: Fetuses born during this period have a fair chance of survival but only with intensive care. They have already acquired some of the necessary immunities and fat for warmth in preparation for life in the outside world. Their nervous system is sufficiently developed for independent functioning. The activity rate of the fetus increases until the final month when the snug fit within the uterus limit is freedom of motion.

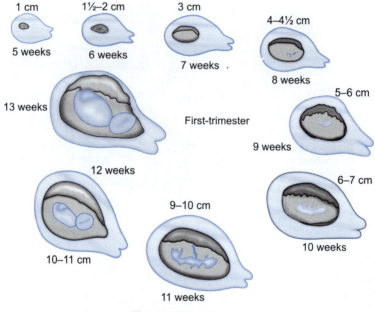

Fig. 20.3 First trimester

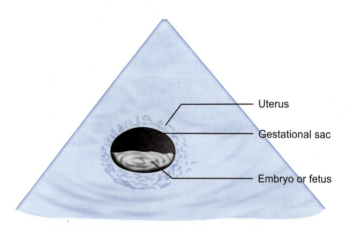

Fig. 20.4 Crown rump length (Transverse section)

The normal period of time required for development of a fullterm fetus is 280 days, although survival is possible after only 180 *in utero*, as mentioned previously (Fig. 20.5).

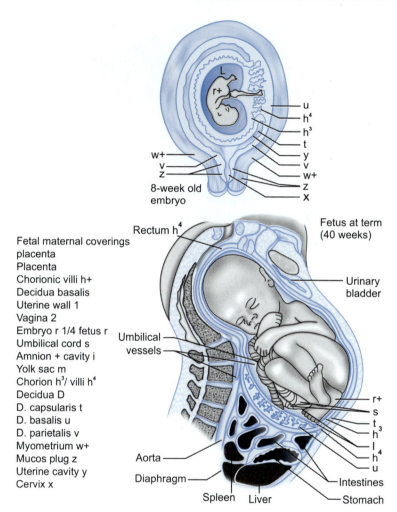

Fig. 20.5 Embryo/fetus

Within the figure:

8-week old embryo

Labels (right of embryo): u, h⁴, h³, t, y, v, w+, z, x

Labels (left of embryo): w+, v, z

Fetus at term (40 weeks)

Rectum h⁴

Urinary bladder

Fetal maternal coverings
placenta
Placenta
Chorionic villi h+
Decidua basalis
Uterine wall 1
Vagina 2
Embryo r 1/4 fetus r
Umbilical cord s
Amnion + cavity i
Yolk sac m
Chorion h³/ villi h⁴
Decidua D
D. capsularis t
D. basalis u
D. parietalis v
Myometrium w+
Mucos plug z
Uterine cavity y
Cervix x

Umbilical vessels

Aorta

Diaphragm

Spleen   Liver

r+, s, t₃, h³, l, h⁴, u

Intestines

Stomach

First Trimester Abnormalities

Ultrasonic diagnostic criteria for a normal first trimester pregnancy are:

- Presence of a well-rounded, intact gestational sac located in the fundus to midportion of the uterus.
- Evidence of embryonic echoes or shadows within the sac by the 6th week.
- Presence of fetal cardiac activity by real-time scan or Doppler, by the 6th week.

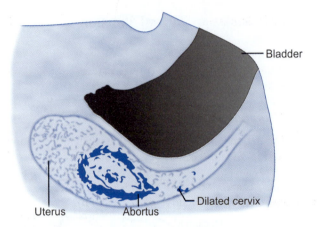

Fig. 20.6 Inevitable abortion (Longitudinal section)

Abnormalities which may be seen during the first trimester listed below. In the presence of these findings, abortion is inevitable (Fig. 20.6).

- Poorly defined or deformed gestational sac (embryonic death/blighted ovum).
- Growth-failure of the gestational sac (embryonic death/blighted ovum).
- Low implantation of the gestational sac with cervical dilatation (inevitable abortion).
- Absence of embryonic echoes or shadows after the 10th week (blighted ovum).
- Absence of fetal heart tones or cardiac motion after the 8th week (fetal demise).

Abortion

It is the term used in obstetrics and gynecology to denote expulsion of product of conception (POC) before the fetus is viable.

Etiology

There is disruption of endometrial tissue due to:

- Genetic defect of embryo
- Hormone levels not adequate to support pregnancy
- External causes (e.g. trauma, viral infection).

There is vaginal bleeding before 20th week with subsequent loss of pregnancy. Abortion occurs in 15% of all pregnancies.

Anembryonic Gestation (Missed Abortion)

Etiology

Clinically the uterus size is less than corresponding dates. Patient's breast tenderness is less.

Ultrasound Findings

Well-formed gestational sac is seen in uterine cavity. No embryo is seen in gestational sac. Size of gestational sac is not appropriate for dates. Transabdominally any sac less than 2.5 cm in diameter, without fetal echoes is an anembryonic gestation. Sometime sac is distorted in shape. It may contain fluid level (due to echogenic blood (Figs 20.7 A and B).

Threatened Abortion

Etiology

Most commonly idiopathic clinical presence of vaginal bleeding (25% cases) and possible mild cramping and backache. Cervix is closed.

Ultrasound Findings

Normal developed gestational sac is seen in uterine cavity, containing an embryo, cardiac pulsations are visible.

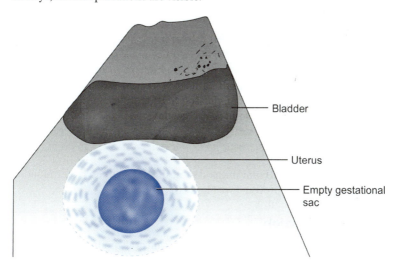

Fig. 20.7A Missed abortion (Transverse section)

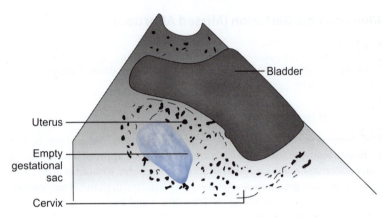

Fig. 20.7B Missed abortion (Longitudinal section)

Crescent-shaped anechoic ring within endometrial canal may be seen. This represents blood outside chorion or amnion.

Incomplete Abortion

Some but not all the product of conception is expelled out. There is persistant bleeding. Cervix is dilated.

Ultrasound Findings

Appearance varies and may include:
- Irregular gestational sac in uterine cavity
- Ill defined echogenic embryo with no cardiac pulsation
- Occassionally clot or decidual tissue may be seen in uterine cavity
- May see dilated cervix
- May see increase corpus luteal flow.

Inevitable Abortion

Persistant bleeding and cramping and some dilatation of cervix. Termination extremely difficult to prevent (*See* Fig. 20.6).

Complete Abortion

Heavy vaginal bleeding is seen. There is expulsion of all product of conception.

Ultrasound Findings

- Normal endometrial canal is seen
- No evidence of intrauterine pregnancy is seen. No product of conception is seen.

Embryonic Demise

Etiology

Nonviable embryo is retained in uterus clinically—no tissue is passed. Patient may or may not bleed. Dropping beta human chorionic gonadotropin (β-hCG) level is seen.

Ultrasound Findings

A gestational sac containing embryo is seen in uterine cavity. No fetal heart rate is seen. Fetus may be small for dates.

Habitual Abortion

Inability of the patient to carry pregnancy beyond a specific point. This inability usually demonstrated several times previously, may occur as a result of an incompetent cervix.

Ultrasound Findings

With a moderate distention of urinary bladder, if cervical length is less than 3 cm, cervical width at internal os is more than 2 cm and cervical canal width is more than 8 mm. This is suggestive of cervical incompetence.

Fetal Circulation

Circulation in the body before birth necessarily differs from circulation after birth for two main reasons:

1. Because fetal blood secures oxygen from the mother's blood instead of from air in the fetal lungs.
2. Because it secures its food from the maternal blood instead of from the fetal digestive organ obviously then, there must be structures to carry the fetal blood into close approximation with the maternal blood and to return it to the fetal body. These structures are the two umbilical arteries, the umbilical vein and the ductus venosus. There must also be some

structure to function as the lungs and digestive organs do postnatally, that is, a place where an interchange of gases, foods and wastes, between the fetal and maternal blood, can take place. This structure is the placenta. The exchange of substances occurs without any actual mixing of maternal and fetal bloods since each flows in its own capillaries.

Since the lungs are functionless before birth, it is not necessary that all blood pass from the right side of the heart to the lungs before reaching the left side of the heart and being pumped to the rest of the body. Therefore, two other structures are present in the fetal circulation, which cease to function at birth and disappear soon after the foramen ovale, an opening in the septum between the two atria, which permits blood to pass directly from the right side of the heart to the left without first going to the lungs: and the ductus arteriosus, a small vessel connecting, i.e. pulmonary artery with the descending thoracic aorta, which permits still more blood to be deflected from the lungs.

In summary, the following structures are essential for fetal circulation but normally cease to exist after birth.

a. Two umbilical arteries, which are extensions of the internal iliac (hypogastric) arteries and carry fetal blood to

b. The placenta, which attaches to the uterine wall

c. The umbilical vein, which returns oxygenated blood from the placenta. The two umbilical arteries and the umbilical vein together constitute the vessels of the umbilical cord, and therefore, are shed at birth along with the placenta.

d. The ductus venosus, a small vessel which connects the umbilical vein with the inferior vena cava (IVC). It closes at birth and disappears soon after.

e. The foramen ovale, an opening in the septum between the right and left atria. Normally it closes at birth. If it fails to close, part of the blood will not be oxygenated and the body's skin will have a bluish color a condition which has led to the term "blue babies."

f. The ductus arteriosus, a small vessel connecting the pulmonary artery with the descending thoracic aorta.

Only two fetal blood vessels carry pure, oxygenated blood; the umbilical vein and the ductus venosus; as soon as the blood enters the IVC it becomes mixed with venus blood.

Ectopic Pregnancy

The word ectopic means 'from location' or 'out of place' and any pregnancy which is not within the uterus is considered ectopic. Extrauterine pregnancies may occur at three sites:

1. In the tube
2. In the ovary
3. In the abdominal cavity.

   Tubal pregnancies occur approximately once in every 100 pregnancies. The tubal pregnancies may occur in the distal or in the mesial or interstitial portion of the tube. Ectopic pregnancy in the distal or ampullary portion will often be expelled into the peritoneal cavity. In this case it is called a tubal abortion. When the pregnancy is halted in the middle third of the tube it will enlarge; the chorionic villi will grow through the wall of the tube where they may penetrate a blood vessel or rupture the tubal wall, causing bleeding into the peritoneal cavity. This results in severe pain, shock from blood loss and some bleeding or spotting from the vagina. This generally occurs 6–12 weeks into the pregnancy. An interstitial ectopic pregnancy is the least frequent, but the most dangerous type, because of the narrowness of the interstitial portion of the tube and its involvement of the uterus. A rupture at this site may involve penetration of large blood vessels or rupture of the uterine cornua causing patient death before surgery can be initiated (Figs 20.8A to C).

   Abdominal ectopic pregnancy occurs rarely and rarest of all are ovarian and cervical ectopic pregnancy. Occasionally an ovum expelled from the tube replants itself in the abdominal cavity and the pregnancy continues to term. In the past, diagnosis was often not made until quite late in this type of pregnancy. Obviously such a pregnancy must be delivered surgically. A serious complication is the removal of the placenta, which usually attaches to the walls of the surrounding intestines.

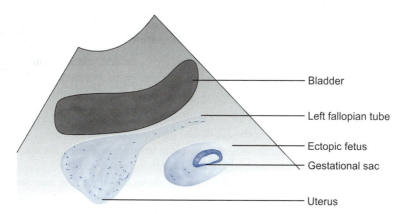

Bladder

Left fallopian tube

Ectopic fetus

Gestational sac

Uterus

Fig. 20.8A Ectopic pregnancy (Transverse section). To diagnose early uterine pregnancy, a double sac sign is visible in ultrasound study

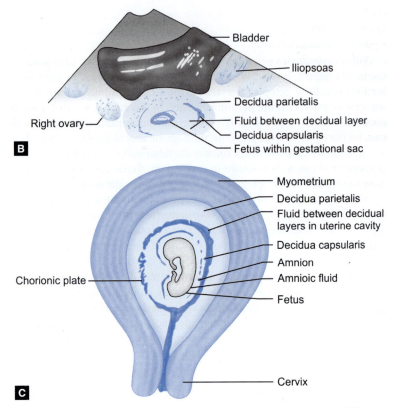

Figs 20.8B and C Double sac sign of early uterine pregnancy (TS)

The diagnostic criteria for ectopic pregnancy is:

- Uterine enlargement (may be only slight, with endometrial thickening).
- Absence of a true gestational sac within the uterus.
- Presence of a primarily cystic or complex appearing structure in the right or left adnexal region or the cul-de-sac (may contain fetal echoes).
- Occasionally in the case of an interstitial or isthmic pregnancy, the cyst-like structure will be seen adjacent to the fundus of the uterus.
- Any ill-defined, anechoic area near or above the umbilicus may be consistent with moderate to massive hemorrhage.

Ruptured tubal/ectopic pregnancy is a more difficult diagnosis to make. This possibility must be considered in the patient who presents with persistent pain, positive pregnancy test, absence of a true gestational sac *in utero* (by ultrasound) and history of a falling hematocrit. Occasionally an extrauterine mass may be seen in the adnexa, containing an increased amount of echoes and possessing less deformed borders than a 'cyst' the exact differentiation between a possible abscess pelvic inflammatory disease (PID) and a ruptured ectopic may be extremely difficult. In case ectopic pregnancy is diagnosed ultrasonologically. The surgery is the only choice of treatment when β-hCG level is below 7000 IU/L. An intrauterine gestational sac is not seen. If any sac structure is seen within the uterus. It is not diagnostically helpful since the differential diagnosis still include a normal or abnormal sac or a decidual cast, laproscopy is helpful.

The failure to identify the intrauterine gestational sac when β-hCG level is above 7000 IU/L indicates that the patient has a very high risk of an ectopic pregnancy and required diagnostic laparoscopy.

In most patients when the β-hCG level is below 7000 IU/L the ultrasound findings are nonspecific. A repeat measurement of β-hCG level after 48 hours is indicated. If β-hCG level is doubled during that interval, a normal pregnancy is suggested.

Classically in ectopic pregnancy there is a decidual reaction (small sonolucent area) within the uterus which may help in diagnosis.

When β-hCG level is above 7000 IU/L a gestational sac should be apparent within the uterus in normal pregnancy.

An intrauterine fetus may be seen before ectopic pregnancy can be excluded. It has been reported that the normal sac can be differentiated because of double echogenic rim.

However, this is of no help in differentiating abnormal aborting sac from decidual casts. The absolute level of serum β-hCG may be very helpful here as well.

Fetal Development

Since amniotic fluid promotes fetal motion, it is important to evaluate fetal position during the ultrasonic examination. The three major positions are:

1. *Cephalic:* In which the fetal head presents at the internal os.
2. *Breech:* In which the fetal buttock presents at the internal os.
3. *Transverse lie:* In which the fetus lies horizontally in the uterus with no major part presenting at the internal os.

   Evaluation of the cephalic presentation may include the position of the fetal head. At first, the ultrasonic appearance of the fetal skull is seen as a relatively circular-shaped structure (8–14th week). As the fetus matures, however, the shape of the fetal skull becomes elliptical or more oval. Careful scanning of the fetal skull will bring out visualization of a strong central midline echo seen to run in the occipitofrontal direction. There is still controversy among investigators regarding the source of this echo. It is most commonly thought to derive from the falx cerebri or the interhemispheric fissure. Whatever the source, the importance of this structure lies in the fact that it provides a landmark toward measurement or an accurate fetal biparietal diameter. When this echopattern is observed it indicates the transducer is level with the brow area of the fetal skull. The true biparietal diameter (BPD) is considered to be the widest transverse diameter perpendicular to the fetal midline echoes, formed by the thalami, peduncles or cavum septum pellucide. Selection of these measurements also depends upon their being equidistant from the anterior and posterior fetal skull vaults. Obviously the most accurate measurements are derived from a fineline depletion of the fetal skull (no more than 3 mm in width).

Ultrasonic instrumentation has made this available by supplying us with the option of leading edge detection in which a preselected, amplitude range discriminates between the strongest echoes and the weakest. Using a measuring device such as electronic or manual calipers, and applying them to the permanent recording of the fetal head scan, the measurement can be calculated.

Once a visually acceptable biparietal is observed and recorded, additional scans should be carried out at 1/2 cm intervals above and below this point to assure that measurement of the widest true diameter of the fetal skull has been obtained.

A helpful aid in scanning the fetus in the cephalic presentation for BPD determination, is the assessment of the angle of asynclitism or the degree of tilt or flexion of the fetal head. The simplest way to do this is to first take a preliminary longitudinal scan to establish the position of the fetal head in relationship to the symphysis pubis. By imagings of the symphysis, an angle is created. After estimating the degree of this angle, the transducer can then be tilted and aligned that same amount and transverse scans are carried out from about 2 cm above the symphysis and upward.

Initially you may wish to actually compute this angle by drawing on the completed record but eventually one learns to gauge this angle visually.

Obtaining a BPD on the fetus in breech presentation is usually more difficult due to the influence of the rising and falling maternal diaphragm on the fetal skull and the range of motion afforded the fetus in this position. This may also hold true with regards to the fetus in transverse lie and it may be necessary to do oblique or tangential scans in this position to achieve access to the occipito frontal areas of the skull. Remember it may be easier to obtain this measurement by emptying the maternal urinary bladder.

The appearance of the fetal skull as a very round structure with only random dots or echoes in the center is a misinterpretation of an adequate biparietal scan. This picture is consistent with a fetal head in the occipital position and only by scanning from an extremely lateral angle can a reliable midline echo complex be elicited. In addition to this ultrasonic picture of an occiput, the presence of echoes derived from the foramen magnum or orbital ridges is also frequently seen. If lateral angles or oblique scans fail to produce a good biparietal measurement. You may wish to try the following:

1. Place the table in modified Trendelenberg's position (15–45°) and rescan.
2. Encourage them to take 10–12 short, panting breaths, with her mouth open, in order to increase the oxygen supply to the fetus and hopefully stimulate it into some movement. Rescan.
3. Empty, or partially empty the bladder and rescan.
4. Turn the patient on other side to encourage a change in fetal position. Resume supine position, and rescan. If none of these techniques is successful, reschedule the patient for re-examination in several days when the fetal position hopefully will have changed (Figs 20.9A to C).

To obtain a biparietal diameter, the sonographer must do three things.

Various charts and graphs have been drived for correlating fetal head size with maturity. One must try to use a chart/graph that most closely approximates the socioeconomic population and geographical features seen in your individual area. If this is not possible, there is a very simple and very general formula which can be adopted. Using a factor of 4, multiply the size

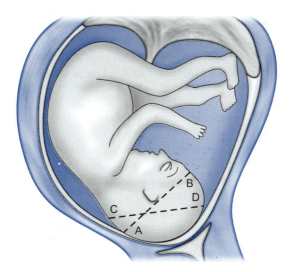

Fig. 20.9A First, find the proper shape, line A-B. Following this axis will give an oval shape. An axis such as C-D will result with an obliques shape

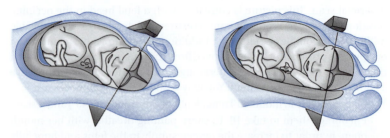

Fig. 20.9B Second, the angle of the transducer to be placed perpendicular to the falx is found. If the transducer is angled too much, or too little, the falx echo will not be equidistant

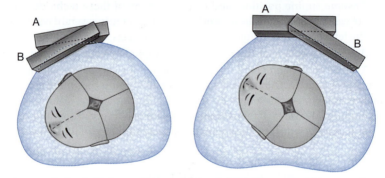

Fig. 20.9C Third, the fetus may have his head tilted down or up. If the transducer is perpendicular to the maternal abdomen, the beam will not be perpendicular to the falx, and only a small portion of the falx echo will be seen. By applying pressure to the end of the transducer that is not perpendicular, the falx echo should come into view

of the fetal skull. The resulting answer approximates the fetal age within 2 week ± its actual age.

In using this formula, some observes feel that the factor should be changed when the fetal head reaches a size greater than 7 cm. At that time they use a factor of 3.8 to allow for the know slow-down in the fetal head growth during the last or third trimester of pregnancy.

The optimum time for obtaining a measurement of BPD between 15 and 26 weeks of gestation. At this stage parameters obtained are influenced mostly by age. After the 26 weeks of pregnancy the measurements are influenced by size as well as age (Figs 20.10 and 20.11).

Other parameters used for estimating gestational age include:

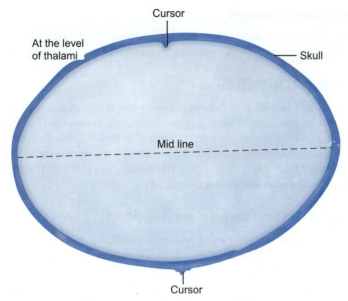

Fig. 20.10 Biparietal diameter (Transverse section)

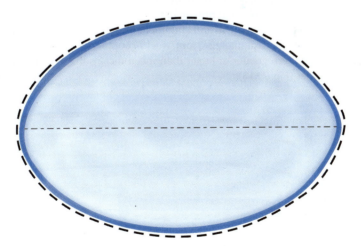

Fig. 20.11 Head circumference (Transverse section)

Femur Measurements

The most accurate time to obtain femur measurement is between 14 and 22 weeks. At this time the measurement is accurate within ± 7 days (Fig. 20.12).

Abdominal Circumference

This can be used where other parameters are not available and offers approximate gestational age. It is not an accurate measurement for dating. An abdominal circumference (AC) measured at the level of left portal vein (umbilical vein), when combined with biparietal diameter is used to obtain an estimated fetal weight. This is useful for relating size to age and also in the diagnosis of intrauterine growth retardation (IUGR) (Fig. 20.13).

Gestational Sac Measurement (Fig. 20.14)

In some cases of IUGR, it is enough to merely measure the fetal head, since this structure may be the last to be affected by the retardation process. It is also necessary to obtain a transverse scan of the fetal abdomen in which vertebral structures and the umbilical vein are demonstrated at opposing ends of the structure. In a normal pregnancy, the fetal head and chest size should be approximately the same. If there is a discrepancy of 1.5 cm or greater, the possibility of IUGR must be considered. It is important to understand that it is not possible to diagnose this condition on the basis of one examination. In interval study, preferably at approximately 3–4 weeks, is necessary to chart the rate of growth of both head and abdomen. It is generally agreed that the fetal head grows approximately 2–3 mm/week or approximately 1 cm/month. Any growth pattern greater or lesser than this indicates the need for serial growth studies (Fig. 20.15).

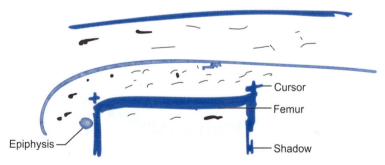

Fig. 20.12 Fetal femur length (Longitudinal section)

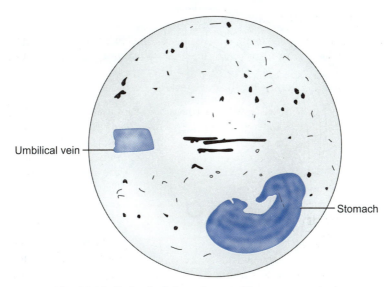

Fig. 20.13 Abdominal circumference (Transverse section)

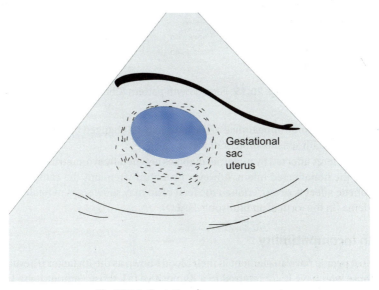

Fig. 20.14 Gestational sac measurement

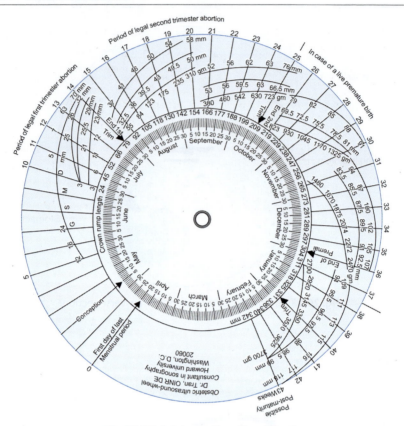

Fig. 20.15 Fetal growth pattern (Chart)

The ultrasonic appearance of the fetus may be changed by the influence of maternal Rh sensitization or diabetes.

The fetus affected by maternal diabetes is generally symmetrically larger than the nonaffected infant, however its maturity remains the same. If the diabetic affect is severe enough the fetal head may show signs of fetal scalp edema (in the form of an ultrasonic HALO).

Rh Incompatibility

Most people have an element in their blood known as the Rh factor (rhesus). Those who have it are referred to a Rh positive (+), those without it are Rh negative (–). The presence or absence of this element itself makes no difference to the health of the individual. It is only when a mother is Rh– and a father is

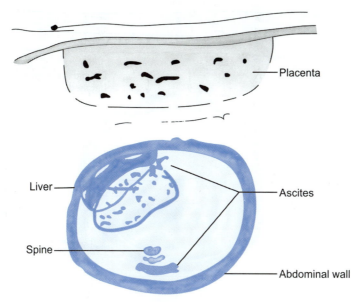

Fig. 20.16 Fetal ascites (Longitudinal section)

Rh+, that blood incompatibility may occur in the unborn child and produce fetal distress or death. Sensitization does not occur in the first pregnancy and it is now medical practice to give Rh negative mothers an injection of Rhogam within 48 hours of birth to block production of antibodies. This agent acts much like a vaccine and eliminates the danger to a future pregnancy. The ultrasonic patterns of RH isoimmunization are generally (Figs 20.16 and 20.17).

1. Larger than average placenta
2. 'Fluffy' appearance of the fetus due to edema
3. Fetal abdominal ascites (in advanced stages)
4. Presence of polyhydramnios, of some degree
5. Abnormal widening of fetal umbilical vein diameter.

Cephalopelvic Disproportion

In the third trimester the clinician may be concerned about the size of the baby's head in proportion to the pelvis of the mother. In a case of this kind the fetal skull should be measured by ultrasound and the maternal pelvis by X-ray pelvimetry.

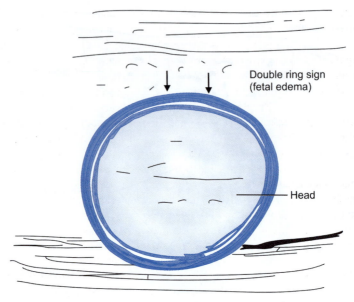

Fig. 20.17 Fetal edema (Transverse section)

Multiple Pregnancy

Twin Pregnancy

The best diagnostic criteria is visualization of two separate fetal bodies and if present, two separate placentae.

In scanning the patient with suspected multiple gestation, it is very important to do not only a complete scan but to extend the parameters of that examination as necessary to cover the entire uterus, in the standard longitudinal and transverse directions and also in the oblique directions. General survey scans are very important. The transverse scan seems to be more helpful in diagnosing the presence of twins, but due to fetal mobility the sonographer should start with longitudinal scans, following established procedure and recording all diagnostic data. As the images are created, it is important to identify each complete fetal structure such as fetal head and thorax, seeing them in their entirety and becoming aware of any additional structure and their locations. Once two fetal heads are identified a mark should be made on the patient's abdomen to locate each of these two structures and a straight line scan made from fetal head-1 to fetal head-2. Generally this will result in the depiction of two fetal heads, obviously separate from one another.

The same procedure may be carried out in identifying and scanning the fetal thoraces and recording their activity by M-mode, real time and Doppler.

An attempt to establish the presence of one or two placentae is also important since if there are two separate placentae we know that the twins are almost always fraternal or nonidentical twins (Fig. 20.18).

The most common combination of fetal position in twin pregnancy are with the lower being cephalic and the upper twin breech or transverse. If both fetuses present in the same direction it is essential to attempt to determine if they are separate from one another. Often the patient is rescanned at a reasonable interval to see if the fetal position have altered. If both fetuses are persistently observed in the same presentation the possibility of Siamese or conjoined twins should be considered. While it is normal for one twin to be slightly larger than the other: it is possible that one twin may develop normally without incidence while the other twin suffers from growth retardation or other complications. Therefore it is necessary that both fetal head/abdomen ratios be obtained and the growth rate of both infants be plotted and compared. If indeed there is failure to grow, on the part of either fetus, amniocentesis is indicated to determine any need for a change in obstetrical management.

One common pitfall in the diagnosis of twins is mistaking a fetal head and chest for two fetal heads, such as seen in transverse lie. Always look for, the known intracranial landmarks that indicate fetal head and for the spinal column that should indicate thorax or abdomen.

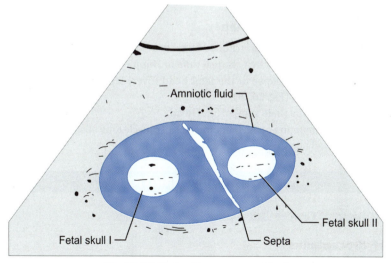

Fig. 20.18 Twins (Transverse section)

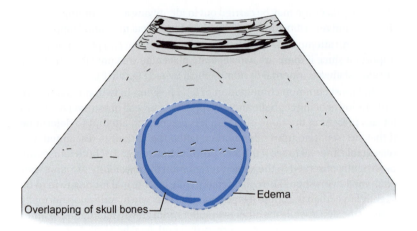

Fig. 20.19 Fetal death-Spalding's sign (Transverse section)

Triplets

Ideally, three fetal heads must be seen in one scan. However, this is seldom the case. Therefore it is necessary to gently, externally, manipulate the fetuses to try to align all three heads in one place and take an oblique scan of them. If this fails you may wish to request this assistance from one of the OB staff.

Complications of Pregnancy

Fetal death: The diagnostic criteria of fetal death are:
- Lack of fetal heart activity by real time or Doppler or M-Mode.
- Deformity or collapse of the fetal head (over) lapping of skull bone-Spalding's sign (Fig. 20.19).
- Double outline (halo sign) of fetal head
- Extreme floatation of the fetus and lack of muscle tone observed as scans are carried out.

FETAL MALFORMATION

Abnormal Cranial Anatomy

Hydrocephalus

One must make comparison of the fetal head and body to indicate significant disproportion. In general, a BPD exceeding 11 cm must be considered

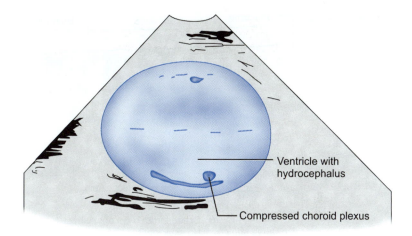

Fig. 20.20 Hydrocephalus

suspiciously hydrocephalic, if the chest size is disparate. Oligohydramnios usually accompanies this condition. In this lateral ventricles are dilated (transverse scan) (Fig. 20.20).

Anencephaly

It is a condition in which well formed fetal skull is absent. The cerebrum, cerebellum and flat bones of skull are generally all absent (Fig. 20.21).

The ultrasonic pattern of anencephaly may reveal no apparent fetal head or else a collection of ill defined echoes in the area in which one would expect to find the fetal head. Polyhydramnios is generally present.

The presence of fetal heart activity will differentiate between anencephaly and fetal death skull deformed. One should scan along the long axis of fetal body to delineate the absence of the head. Usually it is necessary to achieve this scan in oblique fashion. If all efforts to achieve fetal head visualization have failed, one should order an X-ray study for confirmation of ultrasonic study.

Microcephaly

It refers to defective development of cerebrum with a thick skull and early closure of fontanels resulting in a small head. In all of these cases the patient is usually referred for evaluation of a uterus to large for dates. This is usually caused by the presence of polyhydramnios, or excessive amniotic fluid.

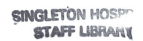

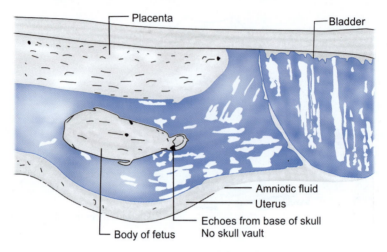

Fig. 20.21 Anencephaly (Longitudinal section)

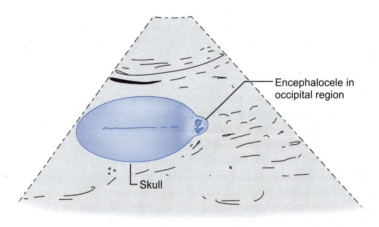

Fig. 20.22 Encephalocele (Longitudinal section)

Encephalocele

In these cases uterus is smaller than the dates. A large cystic mass is noted, projecting from one side of skull wall (Figs 20.22 and 20.23).

The differential diagnosis includes meningomyelocele (continuity with spine) and cystic hygroma.

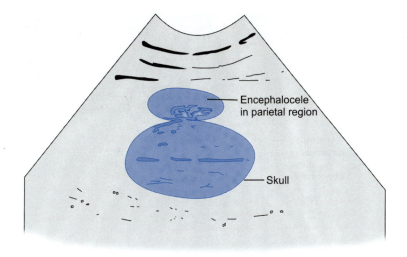

Fig. 20.23 Encephalocele (Transverse section)

When it is associated with infantile polycystic kidneys and growth retardation, Meckel's syndrome should be suspected.

Cystic Hygroma

It is a thin walled multiseptate fluid filled mass, related to fetal neck or head. This mass tends to be asymmetrical. Associated flndings may be fetal ascites and edematous placenta.

Arachnoid Cyst

It is echospared cystic area in the intracranial area. The finding are to be differentiated from porencephalic cyst.

Abnormal Spine Anatomy

Spina Bifida

The fetal spine shows an open wedge shaped defect in longitudinal scan. One can visualize posterior borders of the open spine with protruding meninges (Fig. 20.24).

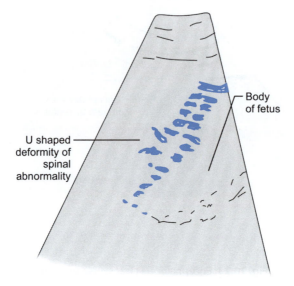

Fig. 20.24 Spina bifida (Longitudinal section)

Meningomyelocele

It can be seen in longitudinal and transverse plane. Posterior border of open spine and protruding meninges and spinal cord is seen (Fig. 20.25).

Abnormal Abdominal Anatomy

Gastroschisis

It consists of a defect in the lateral abdominal wall through which bowel protrudes. It is due to failure in development of small section of the lateral embryonic abdominal wall. Ultrasonologically fetal abdomen with free floating abdominal contents is seen (Fig. 20.26).

Omphalocele

It represents defect in umbilical ring. The herniated contents (intestine, liver, stomach) are contained within a membrane. The umbilical cord enters the defect directly. Polyhydramnios is a frequent finding on these scans (Fig. 20.27).

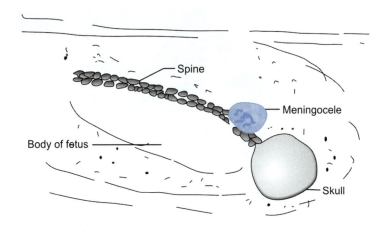

Fig. 20.25 Meningocele (Longitudinal section)

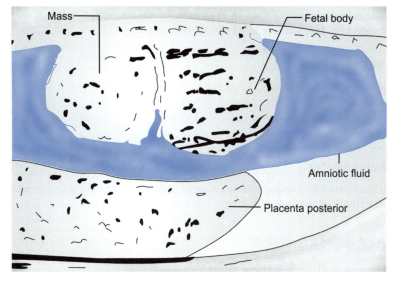

Fig. 20.26 Gastroschisis (Transverse section)

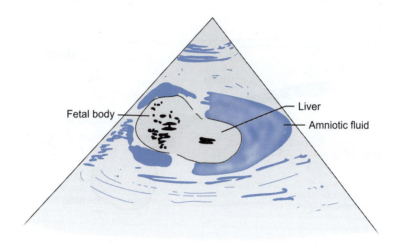

Fig. 20.27 Omphalocele (Transverse section)

Duodenal Atresia

Ultrasonologically it shows double bubble, due to dilated stomach and duodenum. Polyhydramnios is also seen.

Jejunal Atresia

It occurs in approximately 1:350 live births. It is due to mesenteric vascular occlusion.

Dilated bowel loops are visible alongwith polyhydramnios ultrasonologically.

Fetal Ascites

It can be mistaken for hydramnios. Careful scanning at increasing gain should elicit the fetal abdominal outline.

Abnormal Renal Anatomy

Ureteropelvic Junction Obstruction

Longitudinal scan shows dilated renal collecting system. Unilateral/bilateral hydronephrosis is evident. Ureter is not demonstrated. Bladder appears normal.

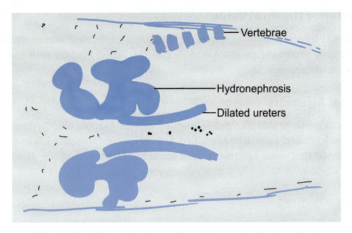

Fig. 20.28 Bilateral hydronephrosis (Longitudinal section)

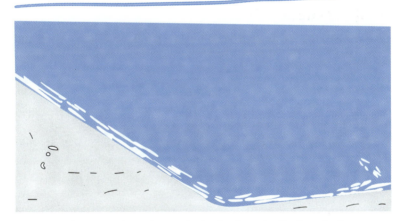

Fig. 20.29 Posterior urethral valve (Longitudinal section)
(markedly distended bladder)

Infantile Polycystic Kidney

It is characterized by large homogenous, echogenic kidneys. No normal anatomy is apparent because of absence of normal renal functions. The bladder is small and there is oligohydramnios.

Posterior Urethral Valve

There is bilateral hydronephrosis. Bladder is distended markedly with distended urethra (Figs 20.28 and 20.29). Thickened bladder wall may be seen in transverse scan.

Renal Agenesis

Patients presents small height of fundus for dates. Marked oligohydramnios is noted. Bladder cannot be identified, kidneys are not visualized. It has been suggested that renal agenesis is best excluded by observing the distended fetal bladder.

CHAPTER 21

Placenta

The placenta is vascular organ developed during pregnancy from the fetal membrane and part of uterine wall. Connected to embryo by umbilical cord, the placenta provides nourishment for fetus, receives and removes fetal wastes and secretes sufficient quantities of progesterone and estrogen in maintenance of gestation.

The placenta can be delineated as early as 10–12 weeks gestation. At this time three areas of placenta can be recognized.

Placental Grading (Fig. 21.1)

Grade 0

Chorionic plate	Straight and well-defined
Placental substance	Homogeneous
Basal layer	No densities

Grade I

Chorionic plate	Subtle undulation
Placental substance	Few scattered echogenic areas
Basal layer	No densities

Grade II

Chorionic plate	Indentation extending into but not to the basal layer
Placental substance	Linear echogenic densities (Comma-like densities)
Basal layer	Linear arrangement of small echogenic areas

Grade III

Chorionic plate	Indentation communicating with basal layer
Placental substance	Circular densities with echo spared areas in center, large irregular densities which cast acoustic shadowing
Basal layer	Large and somewhat confluent basal echogenic areas, can create acoustic shadows.

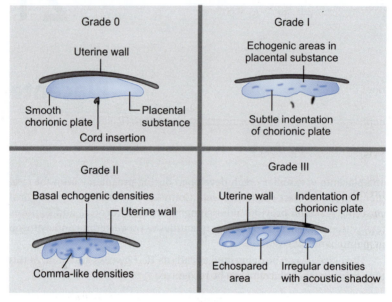

Fig. 21.1 Placental grading

Placenta possesses limited lifespan. It grows and ages, undergoing alteration in structure and function.

Maturation of Placenta

In normal process, the placenta matures, as the gestational age advance.

Grade 0   Up to 30 weeks
Grade I   at 31 weeks
Grade II   36 weeks
Grade III   38 weeks

Premature maturation of placenta is seen in intrauterine growth retardation and in pre-eclamptic toxemia.

Delayed maturation of placenta is seen in Rh sensitized patients and in class I diabetes.

Placental Thickness

Placental thickness seems to decrease as the maturational process progress.

Average thickness of placenta

At	31 weeks	3.8 cm
	35–36 weeks	3.66 cm
	38 weeks	3.45 cm

Placental thickness above 4 cm is seen in class A diabetes Rh sensitized, nonimmune hydropes, thalassemia.

Thin placenta are seen in Juvenile diabetes with retinopathy and nephropathy and in intrauterine growth restriction (IUGR).

Position of Placenta

Placenta can be present in anterior, posterior, fundal, lateral and in placenta previa position (Figs 21.2 to 21.6).

Placental migration: During the second trimester and third trimester placenta is migrated from lower position to upper position of uterus. This is as a result of development of lower uterine segment.

When low lying placenta is seen in second trimester or early third trimester. Repeat the study after two weeks again.

An apparently low position of placenta may be artifactual and depended upon degree of distention of bladder. A repeat scan after voiding demonstrates the true position of placenta. Thus, it is important to rescan the patient after voiding whenever a low placenta is seen.

Multiple Pregnancy

In multiple pregnancy, it is important to note whether there is a single placenta or two placentas. The twins should be evaluated with serial ultrasound profiles every 2–3 weeks. If there are two placentas, the study can be repeated every 4 weeks.

It should be noted that the discrepant growth between the twins with two placentas is still possible, because of local factors, such as abruptio or infarction in one of the placenta (Fig. 21.7).

Placenta Previa

As a condition in which the placenta lies, so low in the uterus that it presents at or encroaches upon the internal cervical os of uterus. Placenta previa is generally classified as follows:

Total previa: Internal os completely covered by placenta (Fig. 21.8).

Partial previa: Partial covering of internal os by placenta.

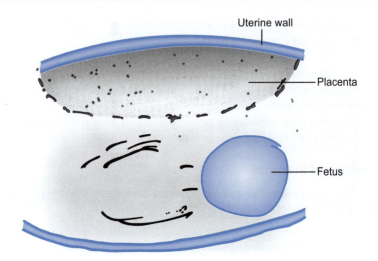

Fig. 21.2 Anterior placenta (Longitudinal section)

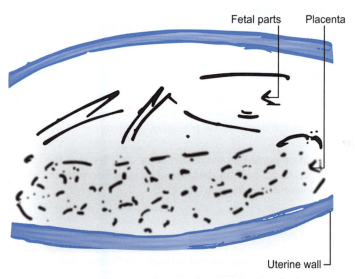

Fig. 21.3 Posterior placenta (Longitudinal section)

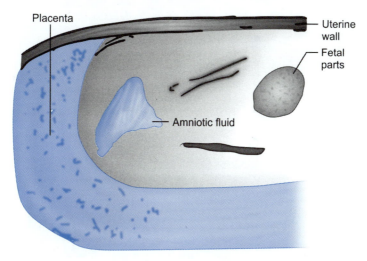

Fig. 21.4 Fundal placenta

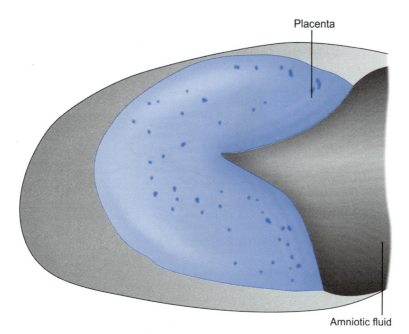

Fig. 21.5 Lateral placenta

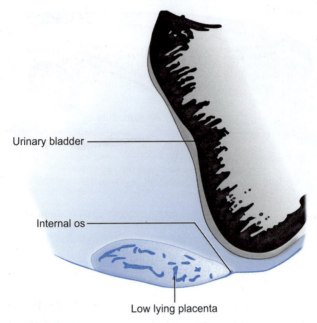

Fig. 21.6 Placenta previa (Longitudinal section) (low lying)

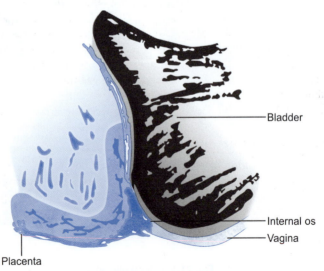

Fig. 21.7 Central placenta previa (Longitudinal section)

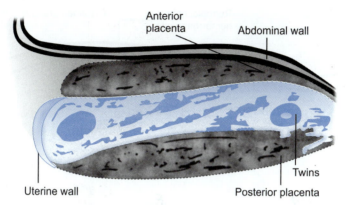

Fig. 21.8 Multiple pregnancies with twin placentas (Longitudinal section)

Marginal previa: Minimal covering of internal os by placenta.

Low lying placenta: A placenta which approximates the internal os but does not encroach upon it.

Ultrasonic evidence of placenta previa is best observed in longitudinal scans in midventral line and with two centimeters to either side of midventral line. Unless the uterus is severely dextrorotated this is the area in which internal cervical os is found. It is absolutely essential that the patient has a well filled urinary bladder. So that area of internal os can be estimated. Care should be taken to avoid over filling of urinary bladder to prevent distortion of lower uterine anatomy which could lead to false impression of placenta previa.

Posterior placenta previa is difficult to diagnose, because fetal cranium causes shadowing across the placenta, making its lower margin difficult to define. In normal, the distance between fetal cranium to the sacrum should not exceed 15 mm. If it exceeds 15 mm it is posterior placenta previa.

Abruptio Placenta

Premature separation of placenta is diagnosed best clinically, based on the symptoms of vaginal bleeding and uterine tenderness. Sometime it is possible to diagnose a retroplacental clot and or retromembranous clot ultrasonographically (Fig. 21.9).

Chorioangioma

They are most common placental tumors.

Placenta demonstrates a subchorionic bulge beneath the insertion of umbilical cord.

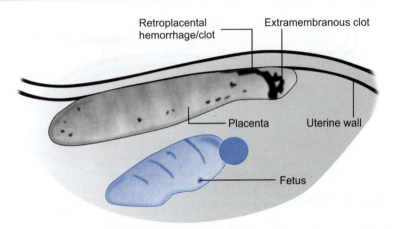

Fig. 21.9 Abruptio placenta (Longitudinal section)

Whenever they are 5 cm in diameter or more they may cause polyhydramnios. There may be onset on premature labor probably secondary to polyhydramnios.

Fetal hypoxia and intrauterine growth retardation may occur because of preferential shunting through the low pressure system of chorioangioma. This hypoxia may increase the frequency of fetal death with large tumors.

Amniotic Fluid

Introduction

The amount of amniotic fluid surrounding the fetus is important during fetal development and affects perinatal outcome.

The amniotic fluid may be normal, decreased (oligohydramnios) or increased (polyhydramnios).

Oligohydramnios

Etiology

   i. Bilateral renal disease
  ii. Intrauterine growth restriction (IUGR)
 iii. Postmaturity
 iv. Premature rupture of membrane
   v. Fetal demise.

Clinically maternal size is small for dates. If oligohydramnios persists for long duration hypoplasia of fetal lungs are seen.

Ultrasound Findings

Largest pocket of amniotic fluid is less than 5 mm.

Fetal extremities are close to body trunk when very less fluid volume and mature placenta are seen before 36 weeks, likely hood of IUGR increases.

Polyhydramnios

Etiology

Increased amniotic fluid is due to fluid secretions and resorption alteration of fetus or mother.

- Idiopathic causes (60% of cases)
- Fetal origin (20% of cases)
  - Neural tube defect
  - CNS defect
  - GI abnormalities
    - i. Tracheoesophageal fistula
    - ii. Esophageal atresia
    - iii. Duodenal atresia
- Maternal origin (20% of cases)
  - Diabetes mellitus
  - Rh incompatibility
  - Multiple pregnancy

Clinically maternal size is larger for dates, may create clinical problems such as premature labor, premature separation of placenta, prolapse cord and postpartum uterine atony.

Ultrasound Findings

1. Excessive amniotic fluid is surrounding the fetus.
2. Fetal extremities seem to float away from body trunk (fetus is swimming) fetus may be normal or there may be neural tube defect, GI defect, congenital heart defect, etc.
3. Multiple fetus may be there.

Assessment of Amniotic Fluid Volume

Amniotic fluid can be evaluated by two methods:
1. Subjectively
2. Objectively with measurements.

Subjective Criteria

Amniotic fluid could be considered normal if it could be demonstrated between fetal limbs and uterine wall anteriorly or between fetal limbs and fetal trunk posteriorly.

Objective Criteria

Studies attempted to quantity amniotic fluid by measuring its largest pocket and setting a lower limit for normal.

1. Manning et al. (1 cm rule) decided that the amniotic fluid could be consider normal if one pocket measures 10 mm or greater in its broadest diameter.
2. Mercer et al defined amniotic fluid as normal if largest pocket was greater than 10 mm size, moderate decrease if pocket was 5–10 mm size and markedly decreased if less than 5 mm.

They found that when cases of ruptured membrane were discarded 7% of neonates with less than 5 mm pocket of amniotic fluid had congenital malformation, increased fetal distress and meconium.

Amniotic fluid assessment

Condition	Single pocket	AFI
Oligohydramnios	< 2 cm	< 7
Reduced	2–3 cm	7–10
Normal	3–8 cm	10–17
More than average	> 8–12 cm	17–25
Polyhydramnios	> 12	> 25

Scan whole uterine cavity for single pocket measure largest vertical pool for amniotic fluid index (AFI) four quadrent method

CHAPTER 23

Assessment of Fetal Wellbeing

Biophysical Profile

Obstetric ultrasound scanning has been used to assess fetal growth parameters that change over relatively long period of time and also to diagnose congenital malformations. Assessing fetal wellbeing on the basis of biophysical parameters such as fetal breathing movements, movements of body and tone has been yet another application of real time ultrasound.

The advantages of high resolution ultrasound imaging is the ability to see the fetus and monitor its activity and responses to a variety of stimuli.

With the introduction of nonstress test (NST), the contraction stress test (CST) to monitor fetus at risk and the concomitant improvement in neonatal care, perinatal mortality has fallen dramatically to less than 12 per thousand live births. The ratio of stillbirth to neonatal death has changed from 1:2 ratio in 1970 to 2:1 in 1980. Thus, prevention of stillbirth has become a major challenge in obstetrics. The causes of stillbirth include chronic intrauterine asphyxia, congenital anomalies and acute complications, e.g. placental methods for the detection of developing fetal asphyxia, if available will reduce both fetal neonatal loss.

Therefore

1. The ideal antepartum test should be highly sensitive and specific.
2. The test should also be capable of identifying a fetus with major anomalies incompatible with intrauterine life and avoiding unnecessary surgical intervention.

Fetal Biophysical Activities

The number of biophysical activities that can be studied by real time B-scan ultrasound are numerous. They include:

1. General biophysical activities such as gross body movement, breathing movement and fetal tone.

2. Specific activities such as sucking swallowing, micturition .
3. Sleep states—recognized by monitoring motion of eyes.
4. Fetal heart rate.
5. Flow in umbilical vessels.
6. The intrauterine environment, in which these activities occur including amniotic fluid volume, placenta grading and pathology and cord position.
7. Evoked fetal reflexes such as startle response.

Factors Affecting Biophysical Activities

The sensitivity of specific central nervous system (CNS) area to hypoxemia is unknown but it has been speculated that variation may exist. The biophysical activities that appear first in fetal development are said to be last to disappear under the influence of progressive asphyxia. When severe enough, causes all biophysical activities to cease.

The absence of fetal tone (which is the earliest to function (7.5–8.5 weeks) is indeed associated with the highest perinatal death rate. On the other hand fetal heart rate reactivity center matures only at about 28 weeks and, therefore, should be more sensitive to asphyxia and should be the first biological activity affected.

The effect on the biophysical profile will depend on the extent, duration, chronicity and frequency of the insult.

With sustained fetal asphyxia, the redistribution of blood to the fetus may lead to reduced or total cessation of perfusion to the lungs and kidneys with decreased urine production and lung liquid flow, resulting in oligohydramnios.

The effects of fetal asphyxia on biophysical variables are of two kinds.

Acute Effects

After an acute insult the fetus shows diminished fetal breathing movements, tone movements and heart rate reactivity (NST).

Chronic Effects

After acute repetitive or chronic asphyxia, the fetus usually shows oligo-hydramnios.

Drugs

CNS-depressors-drugs that depress CNS activity such as sedatives (barbiturates, diazepam), analgesics (morphine) and anesthetics (halothane) usually reduce or abolish fetal biophysical activities.

CNS stimulant and hyperglycemia often result in increased fetal biophysical activities.

Fetal biophysical activities are initiated by complex integrated fetal brain electrical activity, that varies depending on the sleep wake cycle of fetus.

The presence of normal biophysical activity indicates that the portion of CNS that controls the activity is intact and functioning and, therefore, nonhypoxemic.

The absence of a given activity, however is much more difficult to interpret as it may effect either pathological depression or normal periodicity of sleep wake cycles. The periodicity has been shown to be short-term (20–80 minutes) or long-term.

Single Biophysical Variable Tests

Nonstress Test

The combination of fetal heart rate acceleration and fetal body movements has been associated with a high probability of a favorable perinatal outcome. Movements proceedes the onset of most acceleration, indicating some kind of reflex feedback mediated through the neurophysiological pathways initiating the acceleration.

Fetal Movement

i.   *Subjective*: Clinical studies suggesting an association between subjective (maternal) reports of decrease fetal movements and adverse outcome have been confirmed.

ii. *Objective*: These movements can be monitored by real time ultrasound and they occur in episodes of 30 minutes (with 10–16 discrete movements) in each 90 minutes period and appear to be related to sleep wake cycle. There is increase in incidence in inactive fetuses as compared with active one.

iii. *Fetal breathing movements*: The occurrence of rhythmic episodes of breathing movements *in utero* as a part of human fetal development has been documented. Such movements are episodic with burst of fetal breathing interspersed among periods of apnea.

The presence of fetal breathing movements before delivery was a strong predictor of a normal nonstressed fetus (90%); whereas only 50% of fetuses with absent breathing were asphyxiated or depressed at birth.

iv. *Fetal tone*: Hypotonia, characterized by limb deflexion unclasped hands and loss of fist formation, is a natural finding in asphyxiated newborn. Normal fetal tone is defined as active flexion-deflexion of limbs.

Manning suggest this can be assessed equally well by opening and closing of fetal hand.

Fetal tone is considered abnormal, if there is no return to a position of complete flexion after movement or if the fetus is in deflexed position (partial or complete) without movement. Absent fetal tone was associated with a high incidence of fetal distress in labor.

A better objective method of detecting tone is to evoke a fetal startle response with acoustic stimulation.

v. *Placental grade*: Placental grade is not a biophysical variable. It does assess the environment of the fetus.

Patient with grade III placenta had an increased incidence of intrapartum abnormal fetal heart rate pattern and abruptio placentae.

vi. *Amniotic fluid volume*: Decreased AFV, defined as a pocket of fluid less than 1 or 2 cm as seen by real time ultrasound, has been shown to be associated with intrauterine growth retardation and increased perinatal morbidity and mortality. Conditions associated with oligohydramnios are dysmaturity syndrome such as postmaturity, major congenital anomalies mostly involving the genitourinary tract (e.g. renal agenesis).

Composite Fetal Biophysical Variable Monitoring

Since an abnormal test result can be due to asphyxia or the sleep wake cycle. It is necessary to develop a test that can differentiate these two scenarios. This diagnostic dilemma may be resolved by observing multiple biophysical profiles while extending the period of observation beyond a sleep wake cycle.

There are two different kinds of scoring system in the literature:

1. *Manning and associates*: In which variable is scored either normal (2) or abnormal (0) as shown in Table 23.1.
2. *Vintzileos and associates*: In which each variable receives a score of 0, 1 or 2 as shown in Table 23.1.

An Early Predictor of Fetal Infection

Vintzileos and associates suggested that rupture of membranes by itself should not alter the biophysical activity of the healthy fetus (Tables 23.2 and 23.3).

The first manifestation of impending fetal infection were a nonreactive NST and absent fetal breathing. Loss of fetal motion and poor fetal tone were late signs. The presence of fetal breathing had the highest specificity in predicting the absence of infection with no cases of fetal infection when breathing was present 24 hours before delivery.

Table 23.1 Criteria for scoring biophysical variables

Nonstress test	*Score 2 (NST 2):* 5 or more FHR accelerations of at least 15 bpm in amplitude and at least 15 sec duration associated with fetal movements in a 20 min period *Score 1 (NST 1):* 2–4 accelerations of at least 15 bpm in amplitude and at least 15 sec duration associated with fetal movements in a 20 min period *Score 0 (NST 0):* 1 or fewer accelerations in a 20 min period
Fetal movements	*Score 2 (FM 2):* At least 3 gross (trunk and limbs) episodes of fetal movements within 30 min. Simultaneous limb and trunk movements were counted as a single movement *Score 1 (FM 1):* 1 or 2 fetal movements within 30 min *Score 0 (FM 0):* Absence of fetal movements within 30 min
Fetal breathing movements	*Score 2 (FBM 2):* At least 1 episode of fetal breathing of at least 60 sec duration within a 30 min observation period *Score 1 (FBM I):* At least 1 episode of fetal breathing lasting 30–60 sec within 30 min *Score 0 (FBM 0):* Absence of fetal breathing or breathing less than 30 sec within 30 min
Fetal tone	*Score 2 (FT 2):* At least 1 episode of extension of extremities with return to position of flexion and also 1 episode of extension of spine with return to position of flexion *Score 1 (FT 1):* At least 1 episode of extension of extremities with return to position of flexion or 1 episode of extension of spine with return to position of flexion *Score 0 (FT 0):* Extremities in extension. Fetal movements not followed by return to flexion. Open hand
Amniotic fluid volume	*Score 2 (AF 2):* Fluid evident throughout the uterine cavity. A pocket that measures 2 cm or more in vertical diameter *Score 1 (AF I):* A pocket that measures less than 2 cm but more than 1 cm in vertical diameter *Score 0 (AF 0):* Crowding of fetal small parts. Largest pocket less than 1 cm in vertical diameter
Placental grading	*Score 2 (PL 2):* Placental grading 0, 1 or II *Score 1 (PL I):* Placental posterior difficult to evaluate *Score 0 (PL 0):* Placental grading III

Abbreviations: NST, nonstress test; FHR, fetal heart rate; bpm, beats per minute; FM, fetal movements; FBM, fetal breathing movements; FT, fetal tone; AFV, amniotic fluid volumes; PL, placental grading.

Maximal score 12; minimal score 0.

Source: From Vintzileos AM, Campbell WA, Ingardia CJ, Nochimson DJ: The fetal biophysical profile and its predictive value. *Ob Gyn.* 1983;62:271. Reprinted with permission from the American College of Obstetricians and Gynecologists

Table 23.2 Biophysical profile scoring—techniques and interpretations

Biophysical variable	Normal (Score = 2)	Abnormal (Score = 0)
Fetal breathing movement (FBM)	The presence of at least 30 sec of sustained FBM in 30 min of observation	Less than 30 sec of FBM in 30 min
Fetal movements	Three or more gross body movements in 30 min of observation. Simultaneous limb and trunk movements are counted as a single movements	Two or less gross body movements in 30 min of observation
Fetal tone	At least one episode of motion of a limb from a position of flexion to extension and a rapid return to flexion	Fetus is a position of semi-or full-limb extension with no return to flexion with movement. Absence of fetal movement is counted as absent tone
Fetal reactivity	The presence of two or more fetal heart rate accelerations of at least 15 bpm and lasting at least 15 sec and associated with fetal movement in 40 min	No acceleration or less than two accelerations of the fetal heart rate in 40 min of observation
Qualitative amniotic fluid volume	A pocket of amniotic fluid that measures at least 1 cm in two perpendicular planes	Largest pocket of amniotic fluid measures < 1 cm in two perpendicular planes
Maximal score	10	—
Minimal score	—	0

Source: From Manning FA, Morrison 1, Lange IR: Fetal biophysical profile scoring: A prospective study of 1, 184 high risk patients. Am J Obstet Gynecol. 1981;140:289.

Table 23.3 Biophysical profile scoring—management protocol

Score	Interpretation	Management
10	Normal infant, low risk for chronic asphyxia	Repeat testing at weekly intervals. Repeat twice weekly in diabetics and patient ≥42 weeks gestation
8	Normal infant, low risk for chronic asphyxia	Repeat testing at weekly intervals. Repeat testing twice weekly in diabetics and patients ≥42 weeks Oligohydramnios an indication for delivery
6	Suspect chronic asphyxia	Repeat testing in 4–6 hours. Deliver if oligohydramnios present
4	Suspect chronic asphyxia	If ≥36 weeks and favorable then deliver If <36 weeks and L/S <2.0, repeat test in 24 hours. If repeat score ≤4, deliver·
0–2	Strong suspicion of chronic asphyxia	Extend testing time to 120 min. If persistent score ≤4, deliver, regardless of gestational age

Appendix (Fetal Growth)

Clinical parameters in estimation of gestational age*

Priority for estimating gestational age	"Estimated" range for 95% cases
1. *In vitro* fertilization	Less than 1 day
2. Ovulation induction	3–4 days
3. Recorded basal body temperature	4–5 days
4. Ultrasound crown-rump length (CRL)	± .7 weeks
5. First trimester physical examination (normal uterus)	± 1 week
6. Ultrasound BPD prior to 20 weeks	+ 1 week
7. Ultrasound gestational sac volume	± 1.5 weeks
8. Ultrasound biparietal diameter (BPD) from 20 to 26 weeks	± 1.6 weeks
9. LNMP from recorded dates (good history)[†]	± 2–3 weeks
10. Ultrasound BPD 26–30 weeks	+ 2–3 weeks
11. LNMP from memory (good history)	3–4 weeks
12. Ultrasound BPD after 30 weeks	3–4 weeks
13. Fundal height measurement	4–6 weeks
14. LNMP from memory (not good history)	4–6 weeks
15. Fetal heart tones first heard	4–6 weeks
16. Quickening	4–6 weeks

* Rule is to always use a more reliable indicator in preference to a less reliable one.
[†] A "good" history requires knowledge of both last normal menstrual period (LNMP) and previous period with regular periods and no use of birth control pills for at least six months prior to the LNMP.

Fetal crown-rump length against gestational age*

CRL (mm)	−2 SD	Mean weeks	+2 SD	CRL (mm)	−2 SD	Mean weeks	+2 SD
7		6.25	7.15	39	10	10.65	11.35
8		6.45	7.3	40	10.1	10.75	11.45
9		6.7	7.55	41	10.2	10.8	11.55
10	6.25	6.9	7.7	42	10.3	10.9	11.65
11	6.5	7.1	7.9	43	10.4	11.05	11.7
12	6.6	7.25	8.1	44	10.45	11.1	11.8
13	6.85	7.45	8.25	45	10.55	11.2	11.9
14	7.00	7.60	8.45	46	10.66	11.3	12
15	7.15	7.75	8.60	47	10.7	11.35	12.05
16	7.3	7.9	8.70	48	10.8	11.45	12.15
17	7.45	8.1	8.9	49	10.9	11.55	12.25
18	7.60	8.2	9.0	50	10.95	11.6	12.3
19	7.75	8.4	9.15	51	11.1	11.7	12.4
20	7.9	8.5	9.3	52	11.15	11.8	12.5
21	8.05	8.6	9.4	53	11.2	11.85	12.55
22	8.15	8.8	9.55	54	11.3	11.95	12.65
23	8.3	8.9	9.65	55	11.4	12.05	12.75
24	8.4	9.05	9.8	56	11.5	12.1	12.8
25	8.55	9.15	9.9	57	11.55	12.2	12.9
26	8.7	9.3	10	58	11.65	12.3	12.95
27	8.8	9.4	10.1	59	11.7	12.35	13.05
28	8.9	9.5	10.25	60	11.8	12.45	13.15
29	9.05	9.65	10.35	61	11.85	12.5	13.2
30	9.15	9.7	10.45	62	11.9	12.6	13.3
31	9.25	9.85	10.55	63	12	12.65	13.4
32	9.35	9.95	10.65	64	12.05	12.75	13.45
33	9.45	10.05	10.75	65	12.1	12.85	13.55
34	9.55	10.15	10.85	66	12.2	12.9	13.6
35	9.6	10.2	10.95	67	12.3	12.95	13.7
36	9.7	10.35	11.05	68	12.35	13.05	13.75
37	9.8	10.4	11.15	69	12.45	13.1	13.8
38	9.9	10.55	11.25	70	12.5	13.15	13.9

* From Robinson HP, Fleming JEE. A critical evaluation of sonar crown-rump length measurements. Br J Obstet Gynecol. 1975;82:702.

Correlation of predicted menstrual age based upon biparietal diameters

	BPD Mean Values (mm)					
Menstrual age (weeks)	Composite Sabbagha and Hughey[1]	Composite Kurtz et al[2]	Kurtz et al[2] <1974	Kurtz et al[2] >1974	Hadlock et al[3] 1982	Shepard and Filly[4] 1982
14	28	27	28	26	27	28
15	32	31	31	29	30	31
16	36	34	35	33	33	34
17	39	38	39	36	37	37
18	42	41	42	40	40	40
19	45	45	46	43	43	43
20	48	48	49	46	46	46
21	51	51	52	50	50	49
22	54	54	55	53	53	52
23	58	57	58	56	56	55
24	61	60	61	59	58	57
25	64	63	64	61	61	60
26	67	66	67	64	64	63
27	70	69	69	67	67	65
28	72	71	72	70	70	68
29	75	74	75	72	72	71
30	78	76	77	75	75	73
31	80	79	79	77	77	76
32	82	81	81	79	79	78
33	85	83	83	82	82	80
34	87	85	85	84	84	83
35	88	87	87	86	86	85
36	90	89	89	88	88	88
37	92	91	91	90	90	90
38	93	92	92	92	91	92
39	94	94	94	94	93	95
40	95	95	95	95	95	97

1. Sabbagha RE, Hughey M. Standardization of sonar cephalometry and gestational age. Obstet Gynecol. 1978;52:402.
2. Kwtz AB, Wapner RJ, Kurtz RJ, et al. Analysis of biparietal diameter as an accurate indicator of gestational age. J Clin Ultrasound. 1980;8:319.
3. Hadlock FP, Deter RL, Harrist RB, et al. Fetal biparietal diameter: A critical re-evaluation of the relation to menstrual age by means of real-time ultrasound. J Ultrasound Med. 1982;1:97-104.
4. Shepard M, Filly RA. A standardized plane for biparietal diameter measurement. J Ultrasound Med. 1982;1:145-50.

Comparison of predicted femur lengths at points in gestation

Femur Length (mm)				
Menstrual age (weeks)	Filly et al[1] 1981	Jeanty et al[2] 1981[†]	Hadlock et al[3] 1982*	Hadlock et al[3] 1982[†]
12		09	14	08
13		12	16	11
14	16	16	19	15
15	19	19	21	18
16	22	23	23	21
17	25	26	26	24
18	28	30	28	27
19	32	33	30	30
20	35	36	33	33
21	38	39	35	36
22	41	42	38	39
23	44	45	40	42
24	47	48	42	44
25	50	51	45	47
26	53	54	47	49
27	55	57	49	52
28	57	59	52	54
29	61	62	54	56
30	63	65	57	58
31		67	59	61
32		70	61	63
33		72	64	65
34		74	66	66
35		77	69	68
36		79	71	70
37		81	73	72
38		83	76	73
39		85	78	75
40		87	80	76

* Linear function
† Linear quadratic function

1. Filly RA, Golbus MS, Carey JC, et al. Short-limbed dwarfism: ultrasonographic diagnosis by mensuration of fetal femoral length. Radiology. 1981;138:653-6.
2. Jeanty P, Kirkpatrick C, Dramaix-Wilmet M, et al. Ultrasonic evaluation of fetal limb growth. Radiology. 1981;140:165-8.
3. Hadlock Fetal femur length as a predictor of menstrual age: sonographically measured. Am J Roentgenol. 1982;138:875-8.

Head circumference: normal values

Menstrual age (weeks)	Deter et al			Hadlock et al		
	Lower limit* (cm)	Predicted value† (cm)	Upper limit‡ (cm)	−2 SD‖ (cm)	Predicted value§ (cm)	+2SD‖ (cm)
12	5.8	7.3	8.8	5.1	7.0	8.9
13	7.2	8.7	10.2	6.6	8.9	10.3
14	8.6	10.1	11.6	7.9	9.8	11.7
15	9.9	11.4	12.9	9.2	11.1	13.0
16	11.3	12.8	14.3	10.5	12.4	14.3
17	12.6	14.1	15.6	11.8	13.7	15.6
18	13.9	15.4	16.9	13.1	15.0	16.9
19	15.2	16.7	18.2	14.4	16.3	18.2
20	16.4	17.9	19.4	15.6	17.5	19.4
21	17.7	19.2	20.7	16.8	18.7	20.6
22	18.9	20.4	21.9	18.0	19.9	21.8
23	20.0	21.5	23.0	19.1	21.0	22.9
24	21.2	22.7	24.2	20.2	22.1	24.0
25	22.3	23.8	25.3	21.3	23.2	25.1
26	23.4	24.9	26.4	22.3	24.2	26.1
27	24.4	25.9	27.4	23.3	25.2	27.1
28	24.4	26.9	29.4	24.3	26.2	28.1
29	25.4	27.9	30.4	25.2	27.1	29.0
30	26.3	28.8	31.3	26.1	28.0	29.9
31	27.2	29.7	32.2	27.0	28.9	30.8
32	28.1	30.6	33.1	27.8	29.7	31.6
33	28.9	31.4	33.9	28.5	30.4	32.3
34	29.7	32.2	34.7	29.3	31.2	33.1
35	30.4	32.9	35.4	29.9	31.8	33.7
36	31.1	33.6	36.1	30.6	32.5	34.4
37	31.7	34.2	36.7	31.1	33.0	34.9
38	32.3	34.8	37.3	31.9	33.6	35.5
39	32.9	35.4	37.9	32.2	34.1	36.0
40	33.4	35.9	38.4	32.6	34.5	36.4

*   <28 week: Predicted value - 1.5 cm.
    >28 weeks: Predicted value - 2.5 cm.
†   HC = −10.3676 + 1.5021 (MA) −0.0002136 $(MA)^3$ $(R^2 = 97.3\%)$
‡   <28 week: Predicted value + 1.5 cm.
    >28 weeks: Predicted value + 2.5 cm.
§   HC = −10.339 + 1.481 (MA) − 0.0002259 $(MA)^3$ $(R^2 = 98.3\%)$
‖   2 SD = 1.9 cm.

Head circumference: normal values growth rates

Menstrual age interval (weeks)	Deter et al		
	−2 SD[†] (cm/week)	Predicted value* (cm/week)	+2 SD[†] (cm/week)
12–13	1.4	1.6	1.8
13–14	1.3	1.5	1.7
14–15	1.3	1.5	1.7
15–16	1.3	1.5	1.7
16–17	1.3	1.5	1.7
17–18	1.2	1.4	1.7
18–19	1.2	1.4	1.7
19–20	1.2	1.4	1.7
20–21	1.1	1.3	1.5
21–22	1.1	1.3	1.5
22–23	1.2	1.3	1.4
23–24	1.1	1.2	1.3
24–25	1.1	1.2	1.3
25–26	1.1	1.2	1.3
26–27	1.0	1.1	1.2
27–28	1.0	1.1	1.2
28–29	0.9	1.0	1.1
29–30	0.9	1.0	1.1
30–31	0.8	0.9	1.0
31–32	0.8	0.9	1.0
32–33	0.7	0.8	0.9
33–34	0.6	0.8	1.0
34–35	0.5	0.7	0.9
35–36	0.5	0.7	0.9
36–37	0.4	0.6	0.8
37–38	0.4	0.6	0.8
38–39	0.3	0.5	0.7
39–40	0.1	0.4	0.7

* Data represent first derivative values of the function

$$HC = -13.84 + 1.68 \times (MA) - 2.67 \times 10^{-4} (MA)^3$$

which describes the average longitudinal growth curve. These values are calculated as follows:

$$\frac{dHc}{dMA} = 1.68 + 3\,(-2.67 \times 10^{-4})MA^2$$

The values given are mid-week values (i.e. 12–13 week interval: derivative value at 12.5 weeks).

† Values calculated as follows:

$$\left(\begin{array}{l} \frac{2}{9}\left[\sum_{1=1}^{19}\right](a_{11}-1.68)^2 + 9(MA)^4 \\ \times \sum_{1=1}^{19}(a_{3i}+267\times10^{-4})^2 + 6(MA)^2 \\ \times \sum_{1=1}^{19}(a_{1i}-1.68(a_{3i}+2.67\times10^{-4})\frac{1}{2} \end{array} \right)$$

where a_{1i} and a_{3i} are coefficients of the individual HC growth curves.

Abdominal circumference: normal values

Menstrual age (weeks)	Deter et al[13]			Hadlock et al[30]			
	Lower limit* (cm)	Predicted value[†] (cm)	Upper limit[‡] (cm)	−2 SD[‖] (cm)	Predicted value[§] (cm)	+2SD[‖] (cm)
12	5.4	6.3	7.1	3.1	5.6	8.1
13	6.4	7.4	8.3	4.4	6.9	9.4
14	7.4	8.4	9.5	5.6	8.1	10.6
15	8.3	9.5	10.8	6.8	9.3	11.8
16	9.3	10.6	12.0	8.0	10.5	13.0
17	10.2	11.7	13.3	9.2	11.7	14.2
18	11.2	12.8	14.5	10.4	12.9	15.4
19	12.1	13.9	15.7	11.6	14.1	16.6
20	13.1	15.0	17.0	12.7	15.2	17.7
21	14.0	16.1	18.2	13.9	16.4	18.9
22	15.0	17.2	19.5	15.0	17.5	20.0
23	16.0	18.3	20.7	16.1	18.6	21.1
24	16.9	19.4	22.0	17.2	19.7	22.2
25	17.9	20.5	23.2	18.3	20.8	23.3
26	18.8	21.6	24.4	19.4	21.9	24.4
27	19.8	22.7	25.7	20.4	22.9	25.4
28	20.7	23.8	26.9	21.5	24.0	26.5
29	21.7	24.9	28.2	22.5	25.0	27.5
30	22.6	26.0	29.4	23.5	26.0	28.5
31	23.6	27.1	30.6	24.5	27.0	29.5
32	24.6	28.2	31.9	25.5	28.0	30.5
33	25.5	29.3	33.1	26.5	29.0	31.5
34	26.5	30.4	34.4	27.5	30.0	32.5
35	27.4	31.5	35.6	28.4	30.9	33.4
36	28.4	32.6	36.9	29.3	31.8	34.3
37	29.3	33.7	38.1	30.2	32.7	35.2
38	30.3	34.8	39.3	31.1	33.6	36.1
39	31.2	35.9	40.6	32.0	34.5	37.0
40	32.2	37.0	41.8	32.9	35.4	37.9

*   Predicted value −.13 (predicted value).
†   1 AC = −6.9300 + 1.0985 (MA) [R^2 = 95.5%]
‡   Predicted value +.13 (predicted value).
§   1 AC = −10.4997 + 1.4256 (MA) −.00697 $(MA)^2$ [R^2 = 97.9%].
‖   2 SD = 2.5 cm

Ratio of head circumference to abdominal circumference: normal values

| Menstrual age (weeks) | Deter et al | | | Hadlock et al[30] | | | |
	−2 SD [†] (cm)	Predicted value* (cm)	+2 SD [†] (cm)	−2 SD [§] (cm)	Predicted value [‡] (cm)	+2 SD [§] (cm)
12	1.16	1.29	1.41	1.12	1.22	1.31
13	1.15	1.28	1.40	1.11	1.21	1.30
14	1.14	1.27	1.39	1.11	1.20	1.30
15	1.13	1.26	1.38	1.10	1.19	1.29
16	1.12	1.25	1.37	1.09	1.18	1.28
17	1.11	1.24	1.36	1.08	1.18	1.27
18	1.10	1.22	1.35	1.07	1.17	1.26
19	1.09	1.21	1.34	1.06	1.16	1.25
20	1.08	1.20	1.33	1.06	1.15	1.24
21	1.07	1.19	1.32	1.05	1.14	1.24
22	1.06	1.18	1.30	1.04	1.13	1.23
23	1.05	1.17	1.29	1.03	1.12	1.22
24	1.04	1.16	1.28	1.02	1.12	1.21
25	1.03	1.15	1.27	1.01	1.11	1.20
26	1.02	1.14	1.26	1.00	1.10	1.19
27	1.01	1.13	1.25	1.00	1.09	1.18
28	1.00	1.12	1.24	.99	1.08	1.18
29	.99	1.11	1.23	.98	1.07	1.17
30	.97	1.10	1.22	.97	1.07	1.16
31	.96	1.09	1.21	.96	1.06	1.15
32	.95	1.08	1.20	.95	1.05	1.14
33	.94	1.07	1.19	.95	1.04	1.13
34	.93	1.05	1.18	.94	1.03	1.13
35	.92	1.04	1.17	.93	1.02	1.12
36	.91	1.03	1.16	.92	1.01	1.11
37	.90	1.02	1.15	.91	1.01	1.10
38	.89	1.01	1.13	.90	1.00	1.09
39	.88	1.00	1.12	.89	.99	1.08
40	.87	.99	1.11	.89	.98	1.08

*   He/AC = 1.42104 −.0106229(MA) [R^2 = 58.9%].

†   2 SD = 0.12.

‡   HC/AC = 1.32293 −.0084471(MA) [R^2 = 67.2%].

§   2 SD = 0.10.

Mean values for TIUV as a quadratic function of weeks of gestation with upper and lower 2.5 and 10% tolerance limits*

Menstrual weeks	Lower 25%	Lower 10%	Mean	Upper 10%	Upper 2.5%
21	502	789	912	1036	1322
22	507	801	1020	1238	1533
23	536	836	1134	1432	1732
24	589	895	1256	1616	1922
25	667	981	1384	1788	2101
26	771	1091	1520	1949	2269
27	895	1221	1663	2105	2431
28	1033	1364	1813	2262	2593
29	1179	1516	1970	2425	2762
30	1329	1672	2134	2597	2940
31	1483	1832	2306	2780	3129
32	1642	1996	2485	2973	3327
33	1806	2165	2670	3175	3535
34	1980	2345	2863	3381	3746
35	2171	2541	3062	3585	3955
36	2384	2759	3270	3781	4156
37	2623	3004	3484	3965	4346
38	2887	3273	3705	4138	4524
39	3175	3566	3934	4302	4693
40	3484	3880	4170	4459	4855

*From Filly RA. J Clin Ultrasound. 1979;7:24.

Estimated fetal weights (i)*

BPD**	Abdominal circumference

BPD**	15.5	16.0	16.5	17.0	17.5	18.0	18.5	19.0	19.5	20.0	20.5	21.0
3.1	212	219	227	236	244	253	262	272	282	292	303	314
3.2	218	226	234	243	252	261	270	280	290	301	312	323
3.3	225	233	242	250	260	269	279	289	299	310	321	333
3.4	232	241	249	258	268	277	287	298	308	319	331	343
3.5	239	248	257	266	276	286	296	307	318	329	341	353
3.6	247	256	265	274	284	294	305	316	327	339	351	364
3.7	254	263	273	283	293	303	314	325	337	349	361	374
3.8	262	271	281	291	302	312	324	335	347	359	372	385
3.9	270	280	290	300	311	322	333	345	357	370	383	397
4.0	278	288	299	309	320	331	343	355	368	381	394	408
4.1	287	297	308	318	330	341	353	366	379	392	406	420
4.2	296	306	317	328	340	352	364	377	390	404	418	433
4.3	305	315	326	338	350	362	375	388	401	416	430	445
4.4	314	325	336	348	360	373	386	399	413	428	443	458
4.5	323	334	346	358	371	384	397	411	425	440	455	471
4.6	333	344	356	369	382	395	409	423	438	453	469	485
4.7	343	355	367	380	393	407	421	435	450	466	482	499
4.8	353	365	378	391	404	418	433	448	463	479	496	513
4.9	364	376	.389	402	416	431	445	461	477	493	510	527
5.0	374	387	401	414	428	443	458	474	490	507	524	542
5.1	386	399	412	426	441	456	472	488	504	521	539	558
5.2	397	410	424	439	454	469	485	502	519	536	554	573
5.3	409	422	437	452	467	483	499	516	533	551	570	589
5.4	421	.435	449	465	480	496	513	531	548	567	586	606
5.5	433	447	463	478	494	511	528	546	564	583	602	622
5.6	446	461	476	492	508	525	543	561	580	599	619	640
5.7	459	474	490	506	523	540	558	577	596	616	636	657
5.8	472	488	504	520	538	555	574	593	612	633	654	675
5.9	486	502	518	535	553	571	590	609	629	650	672	694
6.0	500	516	533	550	568	587	606	626	647	668	690	712
6.1	514	531	548	566	584	604	623	644	665	686	709	732
6.2	529	546	564	582	601	620	641	661	683	705	728	751
6.3	544	561	580	598	618	638	658	679	701	724	747	772
6.4	559	577	596	615	635	655	676	698	721	744	768	792
6.5	575	594	613	632	653	673	695	717	740	764	788	813
6.6	592	610	630	650	671	692	714	737	760	784	809	835

Contd...

Contd...

	Abdominal circumference											
BPD**	15.5	16.0	16.5	17.0	17.5	18.0	18.5	19.0	19.5	20.0	20.5	21.0
6.7	608	628	648	668	689	711	733	757	780	805	831	857
6.8	626	645	666	686	708	730	753	777	801	827	853	879
6.9	643	663	684	705	727	750	774	798	823	848	875	902
7.0	661	682	703	725	747	771	795	819	845	871	898	926
7.1	680	701	722	745	768	791	816	841	867	894	921	950
7.2	699	720	742	765	789	813	838	863	890	939	945	974
7.3	718	740	763	786	810	835	860	886	913	941	970	999
7.4	738	760	783	807	832	857	883	910	937	966	995	1,025
7.5	758	781	805	829	854	880	906	934	962	991	1,020	1.051
7.6	779	803	827	851	877	903	930	958	987	1,016	1.047	1,078
7.7	801	825	849	874	900	927	955	983	1,012	1,042	1,073	1,105
7.8	823	847	872	898	924	952	980	1,008	1,038	1,069	1,100	1,133
7.9	845	870'	895	922	949	977	1,005	1,035	1,065	1,096	1,128	1,161
8.0	868	893	919	946	974	1,002	1,031	1,061	1,092	1,124	1,157	1,190
8.1	892	918	944	971	999	1,028	1,058	1,088	1,120	1,152	1,186	1,220
8.2	916	942	969	997	1,026	1,055	1,085	1,116	1,148	1,181	1,215	1,250
8.3	941	967	995	1,023	1,052	1,082	1,113	1,145	1,177	1,211	1,245	1,281
8.4	966	993	1,021	1,050	1,080	1,110	1,142	.1,174	1,207	1,241	1,276	1,312
8.5	992	1,020	1,048	1,078	1,108	1,139	1,171	1,203	1,237	1,272	1,307	1,344
8.6	1,018	1,047	1,076	1,106	1,116	1,168	1,200	1,234	1,268	1,303	1,339	1,377
8.7	1,046	1,074	1,104	1,134	1,166	1,198	1,231	1,265	1,300	1,335	1,372	1,410
8.8	1,073	1,103	1,133	1,164	1,196	1,228	1,262	1,296	1,332	1,368	1,405	1,444
8.9	1,102	1,132	1,162	1,194	1,226	1,259	1,294	1,329	1,365	1,402	1,439	1,478
9.0	1,131	1,161	1,193	1,225	1,257	1,291	1,326	1,361	1,398	1,436	1,474	1,514
9.1	1,1'61	1,192	1,223	1,256	1,289	1,324	1,359	1,395	1,432	1,470	1,509	1,550
9.2	1,191	1,223	1,255	1,288	1,322	1,357	1,393	1,429	1,467	1,506	1,545	1,586
9.3	1,222	1,254	1,287	1,321	1,355	1,391	1,427	1,464	1,503	1,542	1,582	1,624
9.4	1,254	1,287	1,320	1,354	1,389	1,425	1,462	1,500	1,539	1,579	1,620	1,661
9.5	1,287	1,320	1,354	1,388	1,424	1,461	1,498	1,536	1,576	1,616	1,658	1,700
9.6	1,320	1,354	'1,388	1,423	1,460	1,497	1,535	1,574	1,614	1,655	1,697	1,740
9.7	1,354	1,388	1,423	1,459	1,496	1,533	1,572	1,611	1,652	1,694	1,736	1,780
9.8	1,389	'1,424	1,459	1,496	1,553	1,571	1,610	1,650	1,691	1,733	1,776	1,821
9.9	1,425	1,460	1,496	1,533	1,571	1,609	1,649	1,690	1,731	1,774	1,817	1,862
10.0	1,461	1,497	1,534	1,371	1,609	1,648	1,689	1,730	1,772	1,815	1,859	1,905

**BPD: Biparietal diameter
* Log (BW)= −1.599 + 0.144(BPD) + 0.032(AC) −0.111(BPD$_2$ × AC)/1,000 SD− +OR −106.0 g per kg of body weight.
Source: Wars of ST, Gohari P, Berkowitz RL, et al. The estimation of fetal weight by computer assisted analysis. Am J Obstet Gynecol. 1977;128:881.

Estimated fetal weights (ii)

BPD**	Abdominal circumference												
	21.5	22.0	22.5	23.0	23.5	24.0	24.5	25.0	25.5	26.0	26.5	27.0	27.5
3.1	325	337	349	362	375	388	402	417	432	448	464	481	498
3.2	335	347	359	372	386	400	414	429	445	461	478	495	513
3.3	345	357	370	384	397	412	427	442	458	475	492	509	528
3.4	355	368	381	395	409	424	439	455	471	488	506	524	543
3.5	366	379	393	407	421	436	452	468	485	503	521	539	559
3.6	377	390	404	419	434	449	465	482	499	517	536	555	575
3.7	388	402	416	431	446	462	479	496	514	532	551	571	591
3.8	399	413	428	443	459	476	493	510	528	547	567	587	608
3.9	411	426	441	456	473	489	507	525	543	563	583	603	625
4.0	423	.438	453	470	486	503	521	540	559	579	599	620	642
4.1	435	451	467	483	500	518	536	555	575	595	616	638	660
4.2	448	464	480	497	514	533	551	571	591	612	633	656	679
4.3	461	477	494	511	529	548	567	587	607	629	651	674	697
4.4	474	491	508	526	544	563	583	603	624	646	669	692	716
4.5	488	505	522	541	559	579	599	620	642	664	687	711	736
4.6	502	519	537	556	575	595	616	637	659	682	706	731	756
4.7	516	534	552	572	591	612	633	655	678	701	725	750	776
4.8	531	549	568	588	608	629	650	673	696	720	745	771	797
4.9	546	564	584	604	625	646	668	691	715	740	765	791	819
5.0	561	580	600	621	642	664	687	710	734	760	786	812	840
5.1	577	596	617	638	660	682	705	729	754	780	807	834	862
5.2	593	613	634	655	678	701	724	749	774	801	828	856	885
5.3	609	630	651	673	696	720	744	769	795	822	850	879	908
5.4	626	647	669	692	715	739	764	790	816	844	872	901	932
5.5	643	665	687	710	734	759	784	811	838	866	895	925	956
5.6	661	683	706	730	754	779	805	832	860	888	918	949	981
5.7	679	702	725	749	774	800	826	854	882	912	942	973	1,006
5.8	698	721	745	769	795	821	848	876	905	935	966	998	1,031
5.9	717	740	764	790	816	843	870	899	929	959	991	1,023	1,057
6.0	736	760	785	811	837	865	893	922	953	984	1,016	1,049	1,084
6.1	756	780	806	832	859	887	916	946	977	1,009	1,042	1,076	1,111
6.2	776	801	827	854	882	910	940	970	1,002	1,034	1,068	1,103	1,138
6.3	797	822	849	876	905	934	964	995	1,027	1,060	1,095	1,130	1,166
6.4	818	844	871	899	928	958	989	1,020	1,053	1,087	1,122	1,158	1,195
6.5	839	866	894	922	952	982	1,014	1,046	1,079	1,114	1,150	1,186	1,224
6.6	861	889	917	946	976	1,007	1,039	1,072	1,106	1,142	1,178	1,215	1,254
6.7	844	912	941	970	1,001	1,033	1,065	1,099	1,134	1,170	1,207	1,245	1,284

Contd...

Contd...

	Abdominal circumference												
BPD**	21.5	22.0	22.5	23.0	23.5	24.0	24.5	25.0	25.5	26.0	26.5	27.0	27.5
6.8	907	936	965	995	1,027	1,059	1,092	1,126	1,162	1,198	1,236	1,275	1,315
6.9	931	960	990	1,021	1,052	1,085	1,119	1,154	1,190	1,227	1,266	1,305	1,346
7.0	955	984	1,015	1,046	1,079	1,112	1,147	1,183	1,219	1,257	1,296	1,337	1,378
7.1	979	1,009	1,041	1,073	1,106	1,140	1,175	1,212	1,249	1,287	1,327	1,368	1,410
7.2	1,004	1,035	1,067	1,100	1,133	1,168	1,204	1,241	1,279	1,318	1,359	1,400	1,443
7.3	1,030	1,061	1,094	1,127	1,161	1,197	1,233	1,271	1,310	1,350	1,391	1,433	1,477
7.4	1,056	1,088	1,121	1,155	1,190	1,226	1,263	1,302	1,341	1,382	1,424	1,467	1,511
7.5	1,083	1,115	1,149	1,184	1,219	1,256	1,294	1,333	1,373	1,414	1,457	1,501	1,546
7.6	1,110	1,143	1,177	1,213	1,249	1,286	1,325	1,364	1,405	1,447	1,491	1,535	1,581
7.7	1,138	1,172	1,207	1,242	1,279	1,317	1,356	1,397	1,438	1,481	1,525	1,570	1,617
7.8	1,166	1,201	1,236	1,273	1,310	1,349	1,389	1,430	1,472	1,515	1,560	1,606	1,653
7.9	1,195	1,230	1,266	1,303	1,342	1,381	1,421	1,463	1,506	1,550	1,595	1,642	1,690
8.0	1,225	1,260	1,297	1,335	1,374	1,414	1,455	1,497	1,541	1,585	1,632	1,679	1,728
8.1	1,255	1,291	1,329	1,367	1,406	1,447	1,489	1,532	1,576	1,621	1,668	1,716	1,766
8.2	1,286	1,323	1,361	1,400	1,440	1,481	1,523	1,567	1,612	1,658	1,706	1,755	1,805
8.3	1,317	1,355	1,393	1,433	1,473	1,515	1,559	1,603	1,648	1,695	1,744	1,793	1,844
8.4	1,349	1,387	1,426	1,467	1,508	1,551	1,594	1,639	1,686	1,733	1,782	1,832	1,884
8.5	1,382	1,420	1,460	1,501	1,543	1,586	1,631	1,676	1,723	1,772	1,823	1,872	1,925
8.6	1,415	1,454	1,495	1,536	1,579	1,623	1,668	1,714	1,762	1,811	1,861	1,913	1,966
8.7	1,449	1,489	1,530	1,572	1,615	1,660	1,705	1,752	1,801	1,850	1,901	1,954	2,007
8.8	1,483	1,524	1,565	1,608	1,652	1,697	1,744	1,791	1,840	1,891	1,942	1,995	2,050
8.9	1,519	1,560	1,602	1,645	1,690	1,736	1,783	1,831	1,881	1,931	1,984	2,037	2,093
9.0	1,554	1,596	1,639	1,683	1,728	1,775	1,822	1,871	1,921	1,973	2,026	2,080	2,136
9.1	1,591	1,633	1,677	1,721	1,767	1,814	1,862	1,912	1,963	2,015	2,069	2,124	2,180
9.2	1,628	1,671	1,715	1,760	1,807	1,854	1,903	1,953	2,005	2,058	2,112	2,168	2,225
9.3	1,666	1,709	1,754	1,800	1,847	1,895	1,945	1,996	2,048	2,101	2,156	2,213	2,270
9.4	1,705	1,749	1,794	1,840	1,888	1,937	1,987	2,038	2,091	2,145	2,201	2,258	2,316
9.5	1,744	1,788	1,834	1,881	1,930	1,979	2,030	2,082	2,135	2,190	2,246	2,304	2,363
9.6	1,784	1,829	1,875	1,923	1,972	2,022	2,073	2,126	2,180	2,235	2,292	2,350	2,410
9.7	1,824	1,870	1,917	1,966	2,015	2,066	2,117	2,171	2,225	2,281	2,339	2,397	2,458
9.8	1,866	1,912	1,960	2,009	2,059	2,110	2,162	2,216	2,271	2,328	2,386	2,445	2,506
9.9	1,908	1,955	2,003	2,052	2,103	2,155	2,208	2,262	2,318	2,375	2,433	2,493	2,655
10.0	1,951	1,998	2,047	2,097	2,148	2,200	2,254	2,309	2,365	2,423	2,482	2,542	2,604

**BPD: Biparietal diameter

* Log (BW) = −1.599 + 0.144(BPD) + 0.032(AC) − 0/111(BPD$_2$ × AC)/1,000 SD= +OR −106.0 g per kg of body weight.

Source: Wars of ST, Gohari P, Berkowitz RL, et al. The estimation of fetal weight by computer assisted analysis. Am J Obstet Gynecol. 1977;128:881.

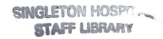

Estimated fetal weights (iii)

BPD**	Abdominal circumference											
	28.0	28.5	29.0	29.5	30.0	30.5	31.0	31.5	32.0	32.5	33.0	33.5
3.1	517	535	555	575	596	617	640	663	687	712	738	765
3.2	532	551	571	591	613	635	658	682	707	732	759	786
3.3	547	567	587	608	630	653	677	701	726	753	780	808
3.4	561	583	604	626	648	672	696	721	747	774	802	831
3.5	579	600	621	644	667	691	715	741	768	795	824	853
3.6	595	617	639	662	685	710	735	762	789	817	847	877
3.7	612	634	657	680	705	730	756	783	811	840	870	901
3.8	629	652	675	699	724	750	777	804	833	863	893	925
3.9	647	670	694	719	744	771	798	826	856	886	918	950
4.0	665	689	713	738	765	792	820	849	879	910	942	976
4.1	684	708	733	759	786	813	842	872	903	934	967	1,002
4.2	703	727	753	779	807	835	865	895	927	959	993	1,028
4.3	722	747	773	801	829	858	888	919	951	985	1,019	1,055
4.4	742	767	794	822	851	881	911	943	976	1,011	1,046	1,082
4.5	762	788	816	844	874	904	936	968	1,002	1,037	1,073	1,110
4.6	782	809	818	867	897	928	960	994	1,028	1,064	1,101	1,139
4.7	803	831	860	890	920	952	985	1,019	1,055	1,091	1,129	1,168
4.8	825	853	881	913	945	977	1,011	1,046	1,082	1,119	1,158	1,198
4.9	847	876	906	937	969	1,003	1,037	1,073	1,109	1,148	1,187	1,228
5.0	869	899	930	961	994	1,028	1,064	1,100	1,138	1,177	1,217	1,259
5.1	892	922	954	986	1,020	1,055	1,091	1,128	1,166	1,206	1,247	1,290
5.2	915	946	978	1,012	1,046	1,082	1,118	1,156	1,196	1,236	1,278	1,322
5.3	939	971	1,004	1,038	1,073	1,109	1,146	1,185	1,225	1,267	1,310	1,354
5.4	963	996	1,029	1,064	1,100	1,137	1,175	1,215	1,256	1,298	1,342	1,387
5.5	988	1,021	1,055	1,091	1,127	1,165	1,204	1,245	1,286	1,330	1,374	1,420
5.6	1,011	1,047	1,082	1,118	1,156	1,194	1,234	1,275	1,318	1,362	1,407	1,454
5.7	1,039	1,074	1,109	1,146	1,184	1,224	1,264	1,306	1,350	1,395	1,441	1,489
5.8	1,065	1,100	1,117	1,175	1,213	1,254	1,295	1,338	1,382	1,428	1,475	1,524
5.9	1,092	1,128	1,165	1,203	1,243	1,284	1,326	1,370	1,415	1,462	1,510	1,560
6.0	1,119	1,156	1,194	1,233	1,273	1,315	1,358	1,403	1,449	1,496	1,545	1,596
6.1	1,147	1,184	1,223	1,263	1,304	1,.;47	1,391	1,436	1,483	1,531	1,581	1,633
6.2.	1,175	1,213	1,253	1,293	1,335	1,379	1,424	1,470	1,517	1,567	1,618	1,670
6.3	1,204	1,243	1,283	1,325	1,367	1,411	1,457	1,504	1,553	1,603	1,655	1,708
6.4	1,233	1,273	1,314	1,356	1,400	1,445	1,491	1,519	1,588	1,639	1,692	1,746
6.5	1,363	1,304	1,345	1,388	1,433	1,478	1,526	1,574	1,625	1,677	1,730	1,786
6.6	1,294	1,335	1,377	1,421	1,466	1,513	1,561	1,610	1,662	1,714	1,769	1,825
6.7	1,325	1,367	1,410	1,454	1,500	1,548	1,597	1,647	1,699	1,753	1,808	1,865

Contd...

Contd...

BPD**	Abdominal circumference											
	28.0	28.5	29.0	29.5	30.0	30.5	31.0	31.5	32.0	32.5	33.0	33.5
6.8	1,356	1,399	1,443	1,488	1,535	1,583	1,633	1,684	1,737	1,792	1,848	1,906
6.9	1,388	1,432	1,476	1,522	1,570	1,619	1,670	1,722	1,776	1,831	1,888	1,947
7.0	1,421	1,465	1,511	1,557	1,606	1,656	1,707	1,760	1,815	1,871	1,929	1,989
7.1	1,454	1,499	1,545	1,593	1,642	1,693	1,745	1,799	1,854	1,912	1,971	2,032
7.2	1,488	1,533	1,580	1,629	1,679	1,730	1,784	1,838	1,895	1,953	2,013	2,075
7.3	1,522	1,568	1,616	1,666	1,716	1,769	1,823	1,878	1,936	1,995	2,055	2,118
7.4	1,557	1,604	1,653	1,703	1,754	1,808	1,862	1,919	1,977	2,037	2,098	2,162
7.5	1,592	1,640	1,690	1,741	1,793	1,847	1,903	1,960	2,019	2,080	2,142	2,207
7.6	1,628	1,677	1,727	1,779	1,832	1,887	1,943	2,001	2,061	2,123	2,186	2,252
7.7	1,665	1,714	1,765	1,818	1,872	1,927	1,985	2,044	2,104	2,167	2,231	2,297
7.8	1,702	1,752	1,804	1,857	1,912	1,968	2,026	2,086	2,148	2,211	2,276	2,344
7.9	1,740	1,791	1,843	1,897	1,953	2,010	2,069	2,130	2,192	2,256	2,322	2,390
8.0	1,778	1,830	1,883	1,938	1,994	2,052	2,112	2,173	2,237	2,302	2,368	2,437
8.1	1,817	1,869	1,923	1,979	2,036	2,095	2,155	2,218	2,282	2,348	2,415	2,485
8.2	1,857	1,910	1,964	2,021	2,079	2,138	2,200	2,263	2,327	2,394	2,463	2,533
8.3	1,897	1,951	2,006	2,063	2,122	2,182	2,244	2,308	2,374	2,441	2,511	2,582
8.4	1,937	1,992	2,048	2,106	2,165	2,226	2,289	2,354	2,420	2,489	2,559	2,631
8.5	1,978	2,034	2,091	2,149	2,210	2,271	2,335	2,400	2,468	2,537	2,608	2,681
8.6	2,020	2,076	2,134	2,193	2,254	2,317	2,381	2,447	2,515	2,585	2,657	2,731
8.7	2,063	2,120	2,178	2,238	2,300	2,368	2,428	2,495	2,564	2,634	2,707	2,781
8.8	2,106	2,161	2,222	2,283	2,345	2,410	2,475	2,543	2,612	2,684	2,757	2,832
8.9	2,149	2,208	2,267	2,329	2,392	2,457	2,523	2,592	2,662	2,734	2,808	2,884
9.0	2,194	2,252	2,313	2,375	2,439	2,504	2,572	2,641	2,711	2,784	2,859	2,936
9.1	2,238	2,298	2,359	2,422	2,486	2,552	2,620	2,690	2,762	2,835	2,911	2,988
9.2	2,284	2,344	2,406	2,469	2,534	2,601	2,670	2,740	2,812	2,887	2,963	3,041
9.3	2,330	2,391	2,453	2,517	2,583	2,650	2,720	2,791	2,864	2,938	3,015	3,094
9.4	2,376	2,438	2,501	2,566	2,632	2,700	2,770	2,842	2,915	2,991	3,068	3,147
9.5	2,423	2,485	2,549	2,615	2,682	2,750	2,821	2,893	2,967	3,043	3,121	3,201
9.6	2,471	2,538	2,598	2,664	2,732	2,801	2,872	2,945	3,020	3,096	3,175	3,256
9.7	2,519	2,583	2,648	2,714	2,782	2,852	2,924	2,997	3,073	3,150	3,229	3,310
9.8	2,568	2,632	2,698	2,765	2,833	2,904	2,976	3,050	3,126	3,204	3,283	3,365
9.9	2,618	2,682	2,748	2,816	2,885	2,956	3,029	3,103	3,180	3,258	3,338	3,420
10.0	2,668	2,733	2,799	2,867	2,937	3,009	3,082	3,157	3,234	3,313	3,393	3,476

**BPD: Biparietal diameter

*Log (BW)= −1.599 + 0.144(BPD) + 0.032(AC) −0.111(BPD$_2$ x AC)/1,000 SD= +OR −106.0 g per kg of body weight.

Source: Wars of ST, Gohari P, Berkowitz RL, et al. The estimation of fetal weight by computer assisted analysis. Am J Obstet Gynecol. 1977;128:881.

Estimated fetal weights (iv)

BPD**	Abdominal circumference												
	34.0	34.5	35.0	35.5	36.0	36,5	37.0	37.5	38.0	38.5	39.0	39.5	40.0
3.1	792	821	851	882	914	947	981	1,017	1,054	1,092	1,131	1,172	1,215
3.2	814	844	875	906	939	973	1,008	1,045	1,082	1,122	1,162	1,204	1,248
3.3	837	867	899	931	965	1,000	1,036	1,073	1,112	1,152	1,194	1,237	1,281
3.4	860	891	924	957	991	1,027	1,064	1,102	1,142	1,183	1,226	1,270	1,316
3.5	884	916	949	983	1,018	1,055	1,093	1,132	1,173	1,215	1,258	1,304	1,350
3.6	908	941	975	1,010	1,046	1,083	1,122	1,162	1,204	1,247	1,292	1,338	1,386
3.7	933	966	1,001	1,037	1,074	1,112	1,152	1,193	1,236	1, 80	1,325	1,373	1,422
3.8	958	992	1,028	1,064	1,102	1,142	1,182	1,224	1,268	1,3 3	1,360	1,408	1,459
3.9	984	1,019	1,055	1,093	1,131	1,172	1,213	1,256	1,301	1,34	1,395	1,445	1,496
4.0	1,010	1,046	1,083	1,121	1,161	1,202	1,245	1,289	1,335	1,382	1,431	1,481	1,534
4.1	1,037	1,074	1,111	1,151	1,191	1,233	1,277	1,322	1,369	1,417	1,467	1,519	1,573
4.2	1,064	1,102	1,140	1,181	1,222	1,265	1,310	1,356	1,404	1,453	1,504	1,557	1,612
4.3	1,092	1,130	1,170	1,211	1,254	1,298	1,343	1,390	1,439	1,489	1,542	1,596	1,652
4.4	1,120	1,160	1,200	1,242	1,285	1,330	1,377	1,425	1,475	1,527	1,580	1,635	1,692
4.5	1,149	1,189	1,231	1,274	1,318	1,364	1,411	1,461	1,512	1,564	1,619	1,675	1,734
4.6	1,179	1,220	1,262	1,306	1,351	1,398	1,447	1,497	1,549	1,603	1,658	1,716	1,776
4.7	1,209	1,250	1,294	1,338	1,385	1,433	1,482	1,534	1,587	1,642	1,693	1,757	1,818
4.8	1,239	1,282	1,326	1,372	1,419	1,468	1,519	1,571	1,625	1,681	1,739	1,799	1,861
4.9	1,270	1,314	1,359	1,406	1,454	1,504	1,555	1,609	1,664	1,721	1,780	1,842	1,905
5.0	1,302	1,346	1,392	1,440	1,489	1,540	1,593	1,647	1,704	1,762	1,822	1,885	1,949
5.1	1,334	1,379	1,426	1,475	1,525	1,577	1,631	1,687	1,744	1,804	1,865	1,929	1,994
5.2	1,366	1,413	1,461	1,510	1,562	1,615	1,670	1,726	1,785	1,846	1,908	1,973	2,040
5.3	1,400	1,447	1,496	1,547	1,599	1,653	1,709	1,767	1,826	1,888	1,952	2,018	2,086
5.4	1,433	1,482	1,532	1,583	1,637	1,692	1,749	1,808	1,868	1,931	1,996	2,064	2,133
5.5	1,468	1,517	1,568	1,621	1,675	1,731	1,789	1,849	1,911	1,975	2,041	2,110	2,181
5.6	1,503	1,553	1,605	1,658	1,714	1,771	1,830	1,891	1,954	2,020	2,087	2,157	2,229
5.7	1,538	1,589	1,642	1,697	1,753	1,812	1,872	1,934	1,998	2,065	2,133	2,204	2,277
5.8	1,574	1,626	1,680	1,736	1,793	1,853	1,914	1,977	2,043	2,110	2,180	2,252	2,327
5.9	1,611	1,664	1,719	1,775	1,834	1,894	1,957	2,021	2,088	2,156	2,227	2,301	2,377
6.0	1,648	1,702	1,758	1,816	1,875	1,937	2,000	2,066	2,133	2,203	2,275	2,350	2,427
6.1	1,686	1,741	1,798	1,856	1,917	1,979	2,044	2,111	2,179	2,251	2,324	2,400	2,478
6.2	1,724	1,780	1,838	1,898	1,959	2,023	2,088	2,156	2,226	2,298	2,373	2,450	2,530
6.3	1,763	1,820	1,879	1,939	2,002	2,067	2,133	2,202	2,273	2,347	2,423	2,501	2,582
6.4	1,803	1,860	1,920	1,982	2,046	2,111	2,179	2,249	2,321	2,396	2,473	2,552	2,634
6.5	1,843	1,901	1,962	2,025	2,090	2,156	2,225	2,296	2,370	2,445	2,524	3,604	2,687
6,6	1,883	1,943	2,005	2,068	2,134	2,202	2,272	2,344	2,419	2,495	2,575	2,657	2,741

Contd...

Contd...

BPD**	\multicolumn{13}{c}{Abdominal circumference}
	34.0	34.5	35.0	35.5	36.0	36,5	37.0	37.5	38.0	38.5	39.0	39.5	40.0
6.7	1,924	1,985	2,048	2,113	2,179	2,248	2,319	2,393	2,468	2,546	2,627	2,710	2,795
6.8	1,966	2,028	2,091	2,157	2,225	2,295	2,367	2,441	2,418	2,597	2,679	2,763	2,850
6.9	2,008	2,071	2,136	2,202	2,271	2,342	2,415	2,491	2,569	2,649	2,732	2,817	2,905
7.0	2,051	2,115	2,180	2,248	2,318	2,390	2,464	2,541	2,620	2,701	2,185	2,871	2,960
7.1	2,094	2,159	2,226	2,294	2,365	2,438	2,513	2,591	2,671	2,754	2,839	2,926	3,017
7.2	2,138	2,204	2,271	2,341	2,413	2,487	2,563	2,642	2,721	2,807	2,893	2,981	3,073
7.3	2,183	2,249	2,318	2,388	2,461	2,536	2,614	2,693	2,776	2,860	2,947	3,037	3,130
7.4	2,228	2,295	2,365	2,436	2,510	2,586	2,665	2,745	2,828	2,914	3,002	3,093	3,187
7.5	2,273	2,342	2,412	2,485	2,559	2,636	2,716	2,798	2,882	2,969	3,058	3,150	3,245
7.6	2,319	2388	2,460	2,533	2,609	2,687	2,768	2,850	2,936	3,023	3,114	3,207	3,303
7.7	2,366	2,436	2,508	2,583	2,659	2,738	2,820	2,904	2,990	3,079	3,170	3,264	3,361
7.8	2,413	2,484	2,557	2,633	2,710	2,790	2,872	2,957	3,044	3,134	3,227	3,322	3,420
7.9	2,460	2,532	2,606	2,683	2,761	2,842	2,926	3,011	3,099	3,190	3,284	3,380	3,479
8.0	2,508	2,581	2,656	2,734	2,813	2,895	2,979	3,066	3,155	3,247	3,341	3,438	3,538
8.1	2,557	2,631	2,707	2,785	2,865	2,948	3,033	3,121	3,211	3,303	3,399	3,497	3,598
8.2	2,606	2,681	2,757	2,836	2,918	3,001	3,087	3,176	3,267	3,360	3,457	3,556	3,658
8.3	2,655	2,731	2,809	2,888	2,971	3,055	3,142	3,231	3,323	3,418	3,515	3,615	3,718
8.4	2,705	2,782	2,860	2,941	3,024	3,109	3,197	3,287	3,380	3,475	3,573	3,674	3,778
8.5	2,756	2,833	2,912	2,994	3,078	3,164	3,252	3,343	3,437	3,533	3,632	3,734	3,838
8.6	2,807	2,885	2,965	3,047	3,132	3,219	3,308	3,400	3,494	3,591	3,691	3,794	3,899
8.7	2,858	2,937	3,018	3,101	3,186	3,274	3,364	3,457	3,552	3,650	3,750	3,854	3,960
8.8	2,910	2,989	3,071	3,155	3,241	3,330	3,420	3,514	3,610	3,708	3,810	3,914	4,021
8.9	2,962	3,042	3,125	3,209	3,296	3,385	3,477	3,571	3,668	3,767	3,869	3,974	4,082
9.0	3,015	3,096	3,179	3,264	3,352	3,442	3,534	3,629	3,726	3,826	3,929	4,035	4,143
9.1	3,068	3,149	3,233	3,319	3,407	3,498	3,591	3,687	3,785	3,886	3,989	4,095	4,204
9.2	3,121	3,203	3,288	3,374	3,463	3,555	3,649	3,745	3,844	3,945	4,049	4,156	4,265
9.3	3,175	3,258	3,343	3,430	3,520	3,612	3,706	3,803	3,962	4,004	4,109	4,216	4,326
9.4	3,229	3,313	3398	3,486	3576	3,669	3,764	3,861	3,961	4,064	4,169	4,277	4,388
9.5	3,283	3,368	3,454	3,542	3,633	3,726	3,822	3,920	4,020	4,123	4,229	4,338	4,449
9.6	3,338	3,423	3,510	3599	3,690	3,784	3,880	3,979	4,080	4,183	4,289	4,398	4,510
9.7	3,393	3,479	3,566	3,656	3,748	3,842	3,938	4,037	4,139	4,243	4,349	4,459	4,571
9.8	3,449	3,535	3,623	3,713	3,805	3,900	3997	4,096	4,198	4,302	4,410	4,519	4,632
9.9	3,505	3391	3,679	3,770	3,863	3,958	4,055	4,155	4,257	4,362	4,470	4,580	4,692
10.0	3,561	3,647	3,736	3,827	3,920	4,016	4,114	4,214	4,317	4,422	4,529	4,640	4,753

**BPD: Biparietal diameter

* Log (BW) = −1.599 + 0.144 (BPD) + 0.032(AC) − 0.111(BPD$_2$ × AC)/1,000 SD= +OR −106.0 g per kg of body weight.

Source: Wars of ST, Gohari P, Berkowitz RL, et al. The estimation of fetal weight by computer assisted analysis. Am J Obstet Gynecol. 1977;128:881.

Index

Page numbers followed by *f* refer to figure

V

W

X